Cast Iron Technology

Volume 2

Brief Contents of

Cast Iron Technology

Volume 1

Volume 2

Cast Iron Technology

Volume 2

Dr S.N. Tiwari

B.Sc. (Met. Engg.), M.Sc. (Met. Engg.), Ph.D. (Met. Engg.)

Director, Moradabad Institute of Technology

Ex-Professor and Head, Department of Metallurgical Engineering, and Ex-Coordinator of Centre of Advanced Study in Metallurgy, Institute of Technology, Banaras Hindu University

Ex-Dean, Faculty of Engineering and Technology, Banaras Hindu University

CBS

CBS PUBLISHERS & DISTRIBUTORS PVT. LTD.

New Delhi • Bangalore • Pune • Cochin • Chennai (India)

ISBN : 978-81-239-1682-8 (PB)
ISBN : 978-81-239-1683-5 (HB)

First Edition : 2009
Reprint : 2012

Published by Satish Kumar Jain and produced by V.K. Jain for
CBS Publishers & Distributors Pvt. Ltd.,
CBS Plaza, 4819/XI Prahlad Street, 24 Ansari Road, Daryaganj,
New Delhi - 110002, India. • Website: www.cbspd.com
e-mail: delhi@cbspd.com, cbspubs@airtelmail.in
Ph.: 23289259, 23266861, 23266867 • Fax: 011-23243014

Branches:

- ***Bengaluru:*** Seema House, 2975, 17th Cross, K.R. Road, Bansankari 2nd Stage, Bengaluru - 560070 Ph.: +91-80-26771678/79 • E-mail: cbsbng@gmail.com, bangalore@cbspd.com
- ***Pune:*** Bhuruk Prestige, Sr. No. 52/12/2+1+3/2, Narhe, Haveli (Near Katraj-Dehu Road By-pass), Pune - 411051 Ph.: +91-20-64704058/59, 32342277 • E-mail: pune@cbspd.com
- ***Kochi:*** 36/14, Kalluvilakam, Lissie Hospital Road, Kochi - 682018, Kerala • Ph.: +91-484-4059061-65 Fax: +91-484-4059065 • E-mail: cochin@cbspd.com
- ***Chennai:*** 20, West Park Road, Shenoy Nagar, Chennai - 600030 Ph.: +91-44-26260666, 26208620 E-mail: chennai@cbspd.com

Printed at :
India Binding House, Noida (UP)

Dedicated
to
My Parents

Preface

Cast irons are the tonnage product of the foundry industry and represent more than 80% of the cast metals produced. Unfortunately, there is hardly any textbook which deals with all aspects of such an important engineering hardware including production technology, metallurgy, properties and applications of all members of a large family of cast irons at one place. The information available in literature is scattered and sometimes confusing and presented in parts in several publications.

It is the endeavour of this author to fill up this existing gap by providing sufficient information on all above aspects of cast irons at one place under the heading *Cast Iron Technology* based on a thorough survey of existing published knowledge, data and information. The author had designed in past a comprehensive course on cast iron technology and has taught different aspects of this course at the undergraduate and postgraduate levels for the last four decades. He is, therefore, hopeful that such a textbook or reference material will be very useful to students and teachers of all the engineering institutions besides the actual plant operators and users of the iron castings.

This book is divided into two parts, Volume 1 and Volume 2, and consists of a total of sixteen chapters. The first part of the book consists of eight chapters dealing with introduction and classification of cast irons, their melting practice with particular reference to developments in cupola melting practice, metallurgy, production technology, characterization and applications of all important family members of cast irons including gray cast irons, white and malleable cast irons, spheroidal graphite cast irons, vermicular (compacted) graphite cast irons and high-duty cast irons. It also provides the relevant references of all the above chapters as a last section of this part of the book.

The second part of this book, Volume 2, also contains eight chapters and deals with the science of production and characterization of special (high-alloy) cast irons, selections of cast irons for different engineering applications, casting defects of iron castings and their remedies, welding of cast irons, inspection and testing of iron castings, design of iron castings as well as their gating and risering design, and finally, the Indian practice of cast iron technology. At the end, it will also include both the subject and the author indexes besides the relevant references of the different chapters.

This book has been also written with a view to encourage advanced research in the areas of cast iron technology by providing the latest available in literature.

Any suggestions by the readers meant to improve the content of this book shall be most welcome and greatly appreciated by the author.

S.N. Tiwari

Acknowledgements

At the outset, I would like to thank the All India Council of Technical Education, New Delhi, for providing me the financial assistance in the form of Emeritus fellowship and the contingency grant to enable me to prepare the required manuscript of this book. It is my duty to express my most sincere thanks and gratitude to all the authors, editors, publishers of the books, monographs, research papers, etc. contained in the 'List of References' whose figures/ photomicrographs have been reproduced and whose work has been frequently consulted and quoted in the compilation of Volumes 1 and 2 of the present book.

I am also thankful to many of my colleagues and friends, particularly Professor S.N. Upadhyaya, Director of the Institute of Technology, B.H.U., and Professor R.C. Gupta, Head of the Department of Metallurgical Engineering, I.T., B.H.U., for encouraging me in this endeavour and providing the library and other departmental facilities and Dr. P. Sriram, my classmate and presently the Joint Managing Director of Rapsree Engineering Industries Ltd., Bangalore, and Shri D.P. Upadhyaya, a very close friend of mine and Ex-Chief Metallurgist, Hindustan Motors, Hoogly, for their guidance and moral support. I am also thankful to one of my students, Shri Upendra Kumar, for helping me in preparing and compiling of the diagrams and photomicrographs as a part of this book. My thanks are also due to Shri Vidya Shankar Singh for his patient and careful typing of the manuscript of this book.

S.N. Tiwari

Contents

9

Special or High-Alloy Cast Irons

9.1 INTRODUCTION

As defined in the chapter 8, SPECIAL CAST IRONS are those irons which have special characteristics, such as high resistance to corrosion, heat or wear, where the enhanced properties are obtained often due to development of special structural constituents by means of additional alloys. These cast irons generally have more than 4% of the alloy content and therefore may also be called as High-Alloy Cast Irons.[61] Various alloying elements are added to the iron for such purposes either singly or in combination such as Ni, Cr, Cu, Mn, Si, Mo, etc. The role of small additions of such elements has been discussed in the previous chapter. However, when nickel is added in higher amounts (3-4%) it tends to produce a micro/constituent namely sorbite (a very fine pearlite) in the matrix and at or more than 5%, it promotes formation of martensite. Above 8% Ni, iron again becomes softer by precipitation of a proportion of austenite and at about 20% Ni, iron is completely austenitic.

On the other hand, chromium acts in opposite to nickel by forming carbides but at the same time, it exerts a grain refining action and thus is similar to nickel in this respect. Nickel and chromium are added singly or together but combination of both is preferred for superior properties as Ni controls chilling and Cr corrects excessive graphitization. Chromium, which is a powerful carbide former also forms complex iron chromium carbides which are more stable than the iron carbide, Fe_3C.

Molybdenum also forms carbide like chromium but is costlier than chromium. It also nodulizes the graphite and promotes formation of a fine pearlite and thus strengthens the matrix.

However, it is used preferably with other elements such as Ni or Cr. Besides nickel, manganese and copper additions also promote formation of austenite. With carbon, manganese also forms stable carbides. The addition of silicon graphitizes the iron and strengthens the ferrite matrix.

Hence, the addition of above alloying elements singly or in combination produces a variety of microconstituents which in turn contribute to the development of special properties of iron suitable for a variety of applications. This chapter, therefore, will be devoted to discussion of these special alloy cast irons with respect to their chemical compositions, microstructures formed, properties developed, and their applications besides the manufacturing process adopted to produce them.

These special cast irons can be classified into two major groups of following high-alloy cast irons.

1. **High-Alloy White Irons** such as Nickel-Chromium White Irons and Chromium-Molybdenum White Irons used for high abrasion and/or wear resistance applications and Special High-Chromium Irons used for corrosion resistance and high temperature service.
2. **High-Alloy Graphitic Irons** such as Austenitic Gray and Ductile Irons and High-Silicon Irons used for high corrosion resistance and heat resistance applications.

9.1.1 Nickel-Chromium White Irons

These irons are low-chromium alloys containing 3 to 5% Ni and 1 to 4% Cr with one exception alloy containing 7 to 11% Cr. These are the oldest group of high-alloy cast irons of industrial importance produced for more than 50 years. Ni-Hard is the trade name of these cast irons which contain hard carbides in a matrix of martensite. These martensitic white cast irons have been developed by International Nickel Limited and are very hard irons used for crushing and grinding parts, for chilled rolls and for sand handling equipment requiring high abrasion resistance. The carbide constituent is harder but more brittle than the martensitic matrix and their combination results in good hardness, abrasion resistance, strength and the toughness required for several applications. Chromium is included in these irons to ensure that the irons solidify carbidic and thus counteracts the graphitic effect of nickel which is responsible for the development of the martensitic matrix.

The Ni-Hard cast irons are produced in four grades,[62] Ni-Hard Type 1 and Ni-Hard Type 2 which are referred to as Standard Grades of Ni-Hard cast irons. Ni-Hard Type 3 is a high-carbon and high-hardness iron whose composition is modified by lowering the carbon content to improve the impact strength of Ni-Hard iron (Table 9.1).

The modified material is known as Ni-Hard Type 2 which has lower amount of brittle carbides leading to improvement in the impact strength with a slight loss in hardness and wear resistance. To improve toughness further, the basic composition of the Standard Ni-Hard is further reduced in carbon content which gives rise to Ni-Hard Type 3 iron. Its draw back is its lower hardness and hence, lower wear resistance.

The failure of Standard Ni-Hard cast irons containing massive carbides results from the initiation and propagation of a crack in the continuous brittle carbide phase formed. Hence, a structure consisting of discontinuous carbide would be advantageous being less susceptible to crack propagation. This principle led to the development of Ni-Hard Type-4 in which a dispersed finer carbide is formed by modifying the composition by increasing the chromium, silicon and nickel contents. The carbides formed in such irons would be in the form of discontinuous chromium carbide $(CrFe)_7C_3$ instead of usual massive continuous carbides, $(FeCr)_3C$. The chromium content of such irons range from 7 to 11% with increased levels of nickel ranging from 5 to 7%. This modification in the pattern of the carbide provides an appreciable improvement in resistance to fracture by impact. The high alloy content of this iron grade also results in improved corrosion resistance which has proved to be useful in the handling of corrosive slurries.

9.1.1.1 Melting, Pouring and Casting Practice

Nickel-Chromium irons can be melted in a cupola but for better control of compositions and temperature, electric melting furnaces such as electric arc melting and induction furnace melting are most commonly used. They are readily made in either acid, neutral or

TABLE 9.1: CHEMICAL COMPOSITION AND MECHANICAL PROPERTIES OF THE NI-HARD ALLOYS [62]

Elements	*Type 1*	*Type 2*	*Type 3*	*Type 4*
Carbon	3.20-3.80	2.80-3.20	2.00-1.60	2.80-3.20
Silicon	0.03-0.50	0.30-0.50	0.40-0.70	1.51-2.00
Manganese	0.30-0.70	0.30-0.70	0.40-0.70	0.40-0.60
Sulphur (Max.)	0.15	0.15	0.50	0.10
Phosphorus (Max.)	0.30	0.30	0.50	0.06
Nickel	3.50-4.50	3.50-4.50	4.00-4.75	5.50-6.50
Chromium	1.50-2.50	1.50-2.50	1.40-1.60	7.00-9.00

Properties	*Sand-Cast*	*Chill-Cast*	*Sand-Cast*	*Chill-Cast*	*Sand-Cast*	*Chill-Cast*	*Sand-Cast*	*Chill-Cast*
Brinell Hardness (Min.)	550	600	525	575	300-500	300-600	550	600
Tensile Strength (psi)	40000-50000	50000-60000	45000-55000	50000-75000	75000-125000	90000-140000	75000 80000	— —
(N/mm^2)	276-345	345-414	310-378	414-516	516-862	621-965	516-552	—
Impact strength (ft./Ib)	20–30	25–40	25–35	35–55	60–70	70–100	25–35	35–55

basic lined electric furnaces. They are normally cold melted. Acid linings are generally more economical than basic linings. Very little adjustments to slag compositions is necessary in acid melting which is used for the majority of current production.

Normal charge materials are various kinds of steel scrap, foundry returns or returns of similar alloy from service. Chromium is obtained in the form of high-carbon ferrochrome and is generally added near the end of the heat to avoid excessive oxidation losses. Carbon is obtained from graphite, petroleum coke and other sources. Silicon and manganese are added as ferro alloys. Molybdenum is usually added as ferromolybdenum.

High superheating temperatures are not necessary when induction melting is used in which good stirring action is achieved and metal is poured at ~1480° C which is adequate for thick-section castings. However, final temperatures of upto 1565° C are commonly used in arc furnace melting to ensure good homogenization of the bath composition and also to accelerate the solution of carbon and late additions. Low pouring temperatures are necessary to avoid problems such as shrinkage defects, metal penetrations and burned-on sand.

Ni-Hard alloys may be sand-cast or chill-cast in permanent moulds. Sand moulds may be made either of green sand, dry sand, oil sand and sands used for steel castings. Air-setting and thermal-setting sands are also commonly used. White irons are subject to hot tearing and suitable precautions are taken to avoid the same during moulding practice. These alloys exhibit relatively high solidification shrinkage and therefore large gates and risers are required for adequate feeding.

9.1.1.2 Heat Treatment

All Ni-Hard white iron castings are given a stress-relief heat treatment since they have a martensitic matrix structure in as-cast condition. Tempering is performed between 205 to 260° C for at least 4 hours. This tempers the martensite, relieves the stresses and increases the strength and impact toughness by 50 to 80%. This heat treatment does not reduce the hardness or abrasion resistance. In the case of low-hardness iron, Ni-Hard Type 4, refrigeration treatment is the more commonly practiced remedy for low hardness achieved. To reduce the amount of retained austenite obtained in as-cast condition and to form more martensite, deep freeze treatments are commonly applied. Refrigeration to temperatures between –70 and –185° C for 1/2 to 1 hour will usually raise the hardness level to 100 HB units. A tempering/stress-relief heat treatment usually follows.

9.1.1.3 Applications

Because of low cost, Ni-Hard cast irons are consumed in large tonnages in mining operations as ball mill liners and grinding balls. Ni-Hard Type 1 castings are used in applications requiring maximum abrasion resistance such as ashpipes, slurry pumps, roll heads, coke-crushers, brick moulds, augers, etc. Ni-Hard Type 2 is recommended for applications requiring more strength and moderate impact such as crusher plates, pulverizer pegs, etc. Ni-Hard Type 4 having high level of strength and toughness is used for more severe applications such as pump whutes and coal pulverizer pegs. Ni-Hard Type 3 is specially designed for production of grinding balls.

9.1.2 Chromium-Molybdenum White Irons

These are high-chromium white cast irons which have excellent abrasion resistance. When the chromium content exceeds 10% level, these cast irons are referred[63] to as high-chromium cast irons and large amount of stable and complex iron-chromium carbides are formed which improve substantially abrasion resistance as well as heat resistance of these irons. These carbides are discontinuous in the structure and this form aids in improving the toughness of the iron.

There are two general classes of the high-chromium irons,[61, 64] the chromium molybdenum irons containing 11 to 23% Cr and up to 3.5% Mo and the second one, containing 23 to 28% Cr with upto 1.5% Mo (Table 9.2). The first grade of these irons are supplied either as-cast with an austenitic or austenitic-martensitic matrix or heat treated with a martensitic matrix microstructure for maximum abrasion resistance and toughness. They are usually considered the hardest of all grades of white cast irons. The second grade of these irons represents the oldest grade of high-chromium irons and are general purpose irons. To prevent pearlite formation and attain maximum hardness, Mo is added in all except the lightest cast-sections. Alloying with Ni and Cu up to 1% is also practiced. The maximum attainable hardness of these irons is not so high as in case of the first grade of Cr-Mo white irons but these alloys are selected when resistance to corrosion is also desired.

9.1.2.1 Melting, Pouring and Casting Practice

The high level of carbon-pickup with the high-chromium contents in these alloys precludes the use of cupola melting. Consequently, electric arc and induction furnaces are frequently used. Acid, neutral or basic-lined electric furnaces are readily adopted for high-chromium iron melting. They are normally dead melted without use of oxygen lancing. Use of acid linings is more economical than basic linings.

TABLE 9.2: TYPICAL COMPOSITIONS AND PROPERTIES OF CHROMIUM-MOLYBDENUM IRONS[61]

Type of Irons	*Composition (%)*						*Properties*
	C	*Mn*	*Si*	*Cr*	*Mo*	*NI*	*(HB)*
11 to 23% Cr-Mo Irons	2.4-3.2	0.5-1.5	1.0 (Max.)	11.0-23.0	1.0-3.5	0.5 (Max.)	450-600
25 to 28% Cr-Mo Irons	2.3-3.0	0.5-1.5	1.0 (Max.)	23.0-28.0	1.5 (Max.)	1.5 (Max.)	400-600

Normal charge constituents are various kinds of steel scrap, foundry returns or similar alloy returns obtained form service. The steel scrap is carefully chosen to ensure that the total content of the alloying elements that affect hardenability and austenite retention is under control. High-carbon ferrochrome is generally added at the end of heat to minimize oxidation losses. Carbon is obtained from different sources such as electrode graphite, petroleum coke, etc. The silicon content of the charge has to be carefully controlled so that it is at the level of 0.6%, as lower silicon content can cause difficulties with viscous slag and high silicon can promote pearlite formation. Manganese should range between 0.5 to 1.5% and Mo is normally added as ferromolybdenum.

High superheating temperatures are not necessary when induction melting is used due to vigorous stirring action available and a pouring temperature of 1480° C is usually adequate. However, higher final temperatures of upto 1565° C are commonly used in arc furnace melting to ensure homogenization of the bath composition and good solution of constituents added after meltdown. Deoxidation of the bath with aluminum is common and Ti is sometimes used to limit dendrite size. Usually, lower pouring temperatures are preferred to have control on feeding problems and other troubles such as penetration and burned-on sand.

Moulds are usually made of either green sand or dry sand, oil sand or sands used for steel casting but they should be rigid to minimize shrinkage defects. Air-setting and thermo-setting resin sands are also used. Precautions are to be taken to minimize hot tearing or cracking as commonly encountered in the castings of white irons or high-chromium irons. Use of cores which break-down easily is preferred. Because of relatively large solidification shrinkage, large gates and risers are required for adequate feeding.

9.1.2.2 Heat Treatment

Toughness and abrasion resistance are improved by suitable heat treatment to get a martensitic structure. Optimum austenitization temperatures are used for achieving maximum hardness such as 955 to 1010° C for irons containing 12 to 20% Cr and 1010 to 1095° C for those containing 23 to 28% Cr. Austenitizing is followed by air quenching to below the pearlite temperature range of 550 to 600° C and then cooling in furnace or still air. However, use of tempering by heating in the range of 205 to 230° C for 2 to 4 hours is recommended to restore some toughness in the martensitic matrix and also to relieve residual stresses. Castings can also be annealed to make them more machinable using annealing or full annealing.

9.1.2.3 Applications

The high-chromium white irons find extensive applications in impellers and volutes, slurry pumps, classifier wear shoes, brick moulds, impeller blades and liners for shot blasting equipment because of their superior abrasion resistance. They withstand heavy impact loading in many applications such as pulverizer rolls, rolling mill rolls, hammers, ring segments in coal grinding mills, etc.

9.1.3 Special High-Chromium Irons

The high-chromium irons in this category have been designed for improved resistance to corrosion for applications such as pumps for handling fly ash and contain 26 to 28% Cr and low-carbon content in the range of 1.6 to 2.0% C. The addition of 2% Mo to these irons is recommended for improving corrosion resistance in the chloride containing environments. Castings are normally supplied in the as-cast condition and the fully austenitic matrix provides the best corrosion resistance though at some loss of abrasion resistance.

There are some high-chromium white iron castings which can be used for intricate and complex parts in high temperature applications at much reduced costs compared to stainless steels. These grades of cast irons have 12 to 39% Cr and can be used for high scaling resistance at temperatures upto 1040° C. The presence of chromium causes the formation of a protective adherent complex oxide film at high temperatures. These high-chromium irons designed for high temperature applications are of following three categories depending on the matrix structures[65]:

1. Martensitic irons with 12 to 28% Cr.
2. Ferritic irons with 30 to 34% Cr as high chromium promotes formation of stable ferrite matrix at room temperature.
3. Austenitic irons which in addition to 15 to 30% Cr also contain 10 to 15% Ni to stabilize the austenite phase.

The carbon content of the above alloys varies in the range of 1 to 2%. Typical applications of these irons are recuperater tubes, breaker bars and trays in sinter furnaces, grates, burners, nozzles and other furnace parts, valve seats for combustion engines, etc.

9.2.1 Austenitic Gray and Ductile Irons

These high-alloy graphitic irons have been developed primarily for applications requiring high corrosion resistance or strength and oxidation resistance in high temperature service (i.e. heat resistance). They are commonly produced in both flake graphite and nodular graphite versions.[66]

These austenitic cast irons, as their name indicates, possess an austenitic matrix, which is stabilized at room temperature by addition of alloying elements like nickel, copper and manganese. Some of these types of irons also contain high proportions of Cr and Si. As such, these cast irons can be broadly classified into three grades namely[67]

1. Ni-Resist Irons
2. High-Manganese Austenitic Cast Irons
3. High-Silicon Austenitic Cast Irons

9.2.2.1 Ni-Resist Irons

These irons include a wide range of austenitic cast irons with nickel contents ranging from 14 to 36%. They include both the flake graphite and spheroidal graphite type. The composition and mechanical properties of the principal grades of these irons are given in Table 9.3. These cast irons are non-magnetic and show high resistance to corrosion by sea water, alkalis, HC1 and H_2SO_4 acids, mine waters, etc. and thus have many applications for pump parts, marine casting, boiler fitting and the like. Among these irons, there is a standard grade and a copper-free grade, the second being used where there is any danger of copper contamination such as food and caustics handling one. Upto 800° C or some what higher, Ni-Resist irons show an excellent resistance to scaling and growth.

9.2.1.2 High-Manganese Austenitic Irons

These irons are also non-magnetic and have a very high specific resistance. This helps in reducing eddy current losses and prevents excessive heating of the electrical machinery. The flake graphite variety of such irons is known as NOMAG and the structure consists of flake graphite and carbide in austenitic matrix. The spheroidal graphite variety of these irons is known as NODUMAG. The main application of these irons is in electrical industry, particularly in power generation equipment and other fields of application include non-magnetic brake drums, electromagnetic devices, signaling systems, clamps in transmission lines, etc. Both flake graphite and spheroidal graphite verities of these irons have essentially similar chemical composition as given in Table 9.3.

9.2.1.3 High-Silicon Austenitic Irons

The flake graphite variety of such irons is known as Nicrosilal and spheroidal graphite variety is known as Spheronic. These irons are used where resistance to high temperature oxidation is required. They are also used for corrosion resistant applications. Higher silicon requires higher nickel to avoid transformation of austenite

TABLE 9.3: COMPOSITIONS AND PROPERTIES OF AUSTENITIC CAST IRONS[68, 69]

Class	*Description*	*Composition (%)*								*Tensile strength*	*BHN*
		C	*Si*	*S*	*P*	*Mn*	*Ni*	*Cu*	*Cr*		
Corrosion Resistant	Ni-Resist (Standard grade)	2.6-3.2	1.0-2.5	0.12 (Max.)	0.40 (Max.)	0.8-1.5	14-17	6-8	1.5-3	10-14 tons/in^2(154-216 N/mm^2)	120-180
	(Cu-Free Grade)	2.6-3.2	1.0-2.5	0.12 (Max.)	0.40 (Max.)	0.8-1.5	18-22	—	1.5-3	10-14 tons/in^2 (154-216 N/mm^2)	120-180
High Electrical Resistant	NOMAG	2.9-3.1	1.5-2.5	—	—	5.5-6.0	10-12	—	—	12-16 tons/in^2 (185-246 N/mm^2)	200-220
Heat Resistant	NICROSILAL A (Hard)	1.9	5.0	—	—	—	18	—	5	16-18 tons/in^2 (246-277 N/mm^2)	320-350
	B (Soft)	1.9	5.0	—	—	—	18	—	2	12-14 tons/in^2 (185-216 N/mm^2)	110-130

to martensite at 600° C resulting in hardness, magnetism and growth. The higher the nickel content, the better is the corrosion resistance whereas the higher the silicon content the better the oxidation resistance.

The flake graphite variety is mainly used for taper plug valves because of its corrosion and heat resistance. The spheroidal graphite variety finds application in furnace parts requiring resistance to oxidation, warping and scaling at high temperatures.

The spheronic type has been successfully used for boxes, trays and baskets and heat treatment furnaces for use upto 900-950° C.

9.2.1.4 Melting, Moulding and Casting Practice

For melting of austenitic cast irons, electric furnaces are exclusively used though in the past cupolas were generally used for this purpose. All kinds of acid, neutral or basic furnace linings are used. Selection of charge materials is more critical particularly for melting of high-nickel alloys of S.G. irons since they are more sensitive to tramp elements present in the charge which may affect the graphite structure. The charge materials are thoroughly dried and melting is fast since presence of nickel in the charge makes it more prone to gas defects. A higher degree of melt super heat is used to take care of temperature losses during melt treatment and pouring is generally done above 1400° C. Magnesium treatment of the base iron is usually done with nickel-magnesium alloys which are often added in the furnace. Foundry grade ferrosilicon containing 75 to 80% Si is commonly added for post inoculation. The latter is performed while tapping the furnace. Besides this, stream inoculation is also recommended for improved machinability.

Sand casting practice including green sand, shell mould and chemically bonded sands is usually adopted. An abrupt change in section thickness should be avoided. Risering is also adopted for feeding purposes. The shrinkage allowances used is of the order of 21 mm/m or 2.10%.

9.2.1.5 Heat Treatment

It is adopted to ensure stability of the microstructure as well as strengthening of nickel-alloyed S.G. iron castings. Stress relieving treatment are usually conducted at temperatures of 620 and 675° C to remove casting stresses. Mould cooling to 315° C is also used as alternative to furnace stress relieving.

Annealing of some castings may be necessary to reduce the hardness and is performed at 955 to 1040° C for 30 minutes to 5 hours. This helps to breakdown some of the carbides formed in the structure and spheroidize the rest. The heat treatment for stability of the microstructure for service at temperatures of 480° C and above is performed by heating at 760° C for a minimum of 4 hours followed by furnace cooling to 540° C and then air cooling. Refrigeration and reaustenitizations are also applied to some alloys to increase the yield strength.

9.2.2 High-Silicon Irons

The high-silicon irons are known by various trade names such as Ironal, Tant Iron, Duniron, Anciron, Corrosion, etc. and are commonly used in the chemical industries for parts where resistance to strongly corrosive liquids coupled with good metallic properties are required. The commercial high-silicon irons are always hypoeutectic in composition and the microstructure consists of α-phase (called as silicoferrite) and fine graphite. In service, a silica like protective film is formed over the casting which inhibits further corrosion. This silica film is not affected by oxidizing, neutral or reducing corrosive agents.

The chemical composition of these alloys falls in the following range[70]:

Carbon	—	0.2 to 0.8%
Silicon	—	13.0 To 18.0%
Manganese	—	0.25 to 1.0%
Sulphur	—	0.05% Max.
Phosphorus	—	0.20% Max.

The properties of these alloys are as follows:

Density	—	6.8 gm/cc
Tensile Strength	—	6 to 7 tons/in^2 (92.4 to 108 N/mm^2)
Compression Strength	—	34 tons/in^2 (523.6 N/mm^2)
Brinel hardness	—	400 to 500

These alloys are used for withstanding corrosive action of H_2SO_4, HNO_3 of all concentrations either cold or hot. Therefore, they are used for equipments handling these acids. They are also used for handling phosphoric acid and NaOH of different concentrations.

The main limitations of these alloys are their tendency to crack down in high temperature applications. They have too low thermal conductivity and therefore their thermal shock resistance is poor. They are brittle alloys at room temperature and therefore careful handling is required.

Table 9.4 shows compositions and provides comparison of general properties of various irons for corrosion resistance applications.

TABLE 9.4: COMPOSITIONS AND PROPERTIES OF CORROSION RESISTANT ALLOY CAST IRON[63]

Composition and Properties	*High-Silicon Irons (Duriron)*	*High-Chromium Irons*	*High-Nickel Irons (Ni Resist)*
% Carbon	0.4-1.0	1.2-2.5	1.8-3.0
% Silicon	14.0-17.0	0.5-2.5	1.0-2.75
%·Manganese	0.4-1.0	0.3-1.0	0.4-1.5
% Nickel	—	0-5.0	14.0-30.0
% Chromium	—	20.0-35.0	0.5-5.5
% Copper	—	—	0-7.0
BHN	450-500	250-400	100-230
Tensile Strength (in 1000 psi)	13-18 (90-124 N/mm^2)	30-50 (270-621 N/mm^2)	25-45 (179-310 N/mm^2)
Charpy Impact (fl.1b)	2-4	20-35	60-150

In sulphur-rich high temperature atmosphere, high-chromium irons are superior to high-nickel and high-silicon irons. However, high-chromium irons compare with high-silicon irons and are complementary to one another in regard to corrosion resistance to nitric acid but are superior to high-silicon irons in regard to mechanical properties. High-Cr irons show excellent corrosion resistance under oxidizing conditions, specially to nitric acid of all concentrations and temperatures upto B.P. for handling of which the high-Si ions are superior. Reducing conditions and the presence of chloride irons and sudden temperature changes may break up the oxide film formed and increase the corrosion rate of high-Cr irons. Therefore, such irons show little resistance to corrosion by HCl and alkalis for which high-Ni irons are better.

9.2.2.1 Melting, Moulding and Casting Practice

Induction melting is the preferred method of melting high-silicon irons.[71] Melting point of eutectic iron of 14.3% Si is about 1180° C and the alloy is generally poured at 1345° C. The charge materials must be carefully controlled to minimize the levels of hydrogen and nitrogen gases. Vacuum melting can be used to increase the strength and density of these alloys.

These alloys are generally cast in sand moulds, investment moulds and permanent steel moulds. Cores used should have good collapsibility to prevent fracture during solidification of these alloys. To avoid cracking, sharp corners and abrupt charges in section size must be avoided. Casting designs should have tapered gates to permit easy removal of gates and risers by impact and to minimize the amount of grinding required. They are usually cast in sections ranging from 4.8 to 38 mm. Casting fluidity of these alloys are good and thin sections can be easily cast.

9.2.2.2 Heat Treatment

High-silicon iron alloys can be stress relieved by heating in the range of 870 to 900° C followed by slow cooling to room temperature to minimize the likelihood cracking. Heat treatments do not affect significantly the corrosion resistance of these alloys.

9.2.2.3 Applications

High-Si irons are mostly used in equipments for production of sulphuric and nitric acids, for sewage disposal and water treatment, for handling of mineral acids in petroleum refining and in manufacture of fertilizers, textiles and explosives.

10

Selection of Cast Irons for Engineering Applications

10.1 INTRODUCTION

In the last few decades, a galaxy of cast irons has been developed, leading to so many types, due to changes in compositions and microstructures and each type of cast iron has some distinguishing property or characteristics and as such is of importance to design and performance in service. The gray cast irons which account for the largest tonnage produced in foundries are of different physical and mechanical properties which can considerably change their service performance and resistance to failure. These differences in properties are caused by the variation in the quantity, shape, size, and size distribution of the graphite flakes formed which in turn are governed by the changes in composition of the iron and rate of solidification and cooling either independently or by combination of the two. It will be an attempt in this chapter to briefly outline the influence of the composition and the microstructures formed on some of the mechanical and physical properties of the service importance before the selection of such cast irons are made for different applications.

The selection of cast irons for different applications is complicated by the combination of the mechanical and physical properties required to withstand service failures due to thermal fatigue, wear and corrosion which may act independently or collectively. However, the selection of gray cast irons will be discussed in respect of a few applications for which such cast iron are well established. Attempt will be also made to recommend cast irons other than gray irons for applications in which inadequate resistance to different types of corrosion and thermal fatigue are the principal causes of failure. Various examples of such cases will be presented to highlight the need for carefully analyzing the service requirements for proper selection of the meterial.

10.2 EFFECT OF COMPOSITION AND STRUCTURE ON DIFFERENT PROPERTIES OF CAST IRONS

The following are the general observations[72-76] of the effects of composition and microstructure on some of the important mechanical, physical and service properties of cast irons which will have considerable impact on the design and performance of many different types of general engineering components:

10.2.1 Mechanical Properties

1. Tensile strength of cast irons increases with change in the shape of graphite from flake to some kind of aggregates of graphite like temper carbon in malleable irons and spherical graphite in S.G. cast irons, which causes least interruption to the continuity of the metallic matrix. This change in shape of graphite also improves the ductility of the iron for the same reason.
2. Tensile strength is also influenced by the nature of the matrix. A fine and fully pearlitic matrix increases the strength and hardness together with good machinability.
3. Cementite in the matrix increases hardness and wear resistance at the expense of the toughness and machinability while ferrite increases toughness and ductility at the expense of strength, hardness and wear resistance.
4. In case of malleable and S.G. irons, tensile properties are mainly controlled by the matrix structure whereas the quantity, shape and size of the graphite flakes chiefly control the tensile strength of the gray irons.
5. The carbon equivalent and the cooling rate as influenced by the section size control the quantity of graphite in the matrix structure of the gray irons and therefore, they affect considerably the strength properties.
6. In case of malleable and S.G. irons, the elastic modulus is not influenced by the nature of the matrix and remains virtually constant and does not vary with the tensile

strength, where as in the gray irons the quantity, shape and size of graphite affect the elastic modulus as they also affect the strength of the iron.

7. Hardness is normally directly related to strength in many cast irons but in gray irons, the size, shape and quantity of graphite flakes present as well as the cementite and the phosphide eutectic formed in the structure interfere with such relation.
8. Fatigue properties are governed jointly by the endurance limit and the notch sensitivity of the material. The endurance limit bear a direct ratio to tensile strength for each class of the material and hence, the microstructure and composition affect this property in the same way as the strength. The gray irons have the lowest notch sensitivity of all irons because of the flake shapes of graphite present in the structure.

10.2.2 Physical Properties

1. Gray cast irons have excellent damping capacity due to the flake shape of the graphite. Damping capacity varies approximately inversely with the elastic modulus of the meterial.
2. Thermal conductivity of different cast irons is governed primarily by the quantity and the shape of the graphite present and the nature of the matrix formed. Hence, highest thermal conductivity is associated with flake graphite types of irons having a high quantity of the graphite. A high total carbon and high carbon equivalence increase thermal conductivity in gray cast irons. As the graphite becomes spheroidal and the matrix changes from ferrite to austenite the thermal conductivity is significantly reduced.
3. The thermal expansion characteristics of irons having a ferrite or pearlitic matrix do not change with the matrix. However, when matrix changes to austenite thermal characteristics vary widely.

10.2.3 Service Properties

1. Various properties like wear and abrasion resistance, corrosion resistance and heat resistance fall under the

category of service properties. In general, cast irons have superior wear resistance compared to steel. Under sliding conditions, gray cast irons having greater graphite quantity of medium coarseness have good wear resistance. The presence of ferrite in the matrix decreases wear resistance whereas a well dispersed carbide/phosphide eutectic is beneficial for wear resistance.

2. Under abrasive wear conditions, a carbide-containing iron having a martensitic matrix such as Ni-Hard gives outstanding wear resistance. A good surface finish prevents wear by promoting conditions of hydrodynamic lubrication.
3. The common causes of failure due to rise in the temperature of a component are thermal shock and oxidation characteristics and growth of the material. Thermal shock is caused by alternate heating and cooling which setup residual stresses. The alloy gray cast irons in general and of the nickel-containing types in particular, have superior thermal shock resistance.
4. A structurally stabler gray iron will not undergo growth upto the transformations temperature. Use of high alloy irons like austenitic types or high-chromium or high-silicon types have better resistance to growth and oxidation.
5. The additions of Cr, Si and Ni improve the corrosion resistance of gray irons by forming stable and tenacious oxide films on the surface of the casting. In sulphur-rich high temperature atmosphere, high-chromium irons are superior to high-silicon and high-nickel irons in improving the corrosion resistance. High-Cr irons show excellent corrosion resistance under oxidizing conditions. Under reducing conditions and in the presence of chloride ions, high-Cr irons show little resistance to corrosion for which high-Ni irons are better.
6. In high-Cr irons, large amount of stable complex iron-chromium carbides are formed which improve the abrasion resistance as well as heat resistance of these irons.

10.3 SELECTION OF CAST IRONS FOR DIFFERENT APPLICATIONS

The choice of cast irons for different applications is complicated by conflicting nature of different property requirements posed by the service condition. However, for a satisfactory performance of a meterial, the selection should be based on an optimum combination of other properties in relation to the main property required to avoid the service failure of the component.

Some of the typical engineering applications for which selection of different cast irons is made will be illustrated in this section as examples and they are by no means exhaustive and are intended to convey the need for careful analysis of the service requirement before the selection is made.

10.3.1 Machine Tool Slide Ways and Cylinder Liners

For these applications, the principal meterial characteristics is the resistance to wear under a lubricated reciprocating sliding condition and the gray cast iron is the meterial which is mostly used.This type of the wear involves metal-to-metal contact leading to both the adhesive and abrasive wear. The extent of the latter increases depending upon the degree of contamination of the oil film from different sources. In the case of machine tool slide ways, this contamination is derived from the dust formed during the grinding operation or from the chips and dust formed during machining the cast iron. In the case of cylinder liners, contamination arises from dirt and debris carried with the oil and from the carbon deposits or ash produced from the fuel and the lubricating oils. The fretting corrosion in the case of machine tool sideways and the corrosion by the products of combustion and moisture condensation in the case of cylinder liners further aggravate this wear.

Several investigations of wear of machine tool slide ways have recommended use of gray iron with high carbon content (> 3.2%C) with medium to coarse graphite flakes of Type A and a high phosphorus content of 0.7 to 1.4% together with low silicon as the most desirable component material. A hardness of 180-240 BHN is satisfactory and in the absense of or with low value of phosphorus, a fully pearlitic matrix is desirable. A higher hardness will be necessary as the extent of abrasive wear increases. The surface hardening treatment of the slide ways is recommended under such conditions. The presence of alloying elements such as Ni (0.8 to 1%) and Cr (0.3 to 0.5) in the iron will give the best results.

The above specifications of the material will also be suitable for cylinder liners. However, these components are centrifugally cast and it may not be possible to maintain a uniform shape of the graphite through out the casting. It is advocated to limit the phosphorus content of iron to < 0.2% because of the tendency to form pinholes when phosphorus is high. Under such conditions, to limit the formation of ferrite, additions of vanadium to iron is recommended which will promote formation of a well dispersed carbide/phosphide eutectic. Oil quenching of the cylinder liners of such iron will increase the hardness desirable under abrasive wear conditions.

10.3.2 Brake Drums and Cylinder Heads

The main cause of service failure of the above components for which gray cast iron is predominantly used is thermal cracking and therefore the latter is the prime consideration for selection of the material.

The amount of heat generated in a brake drum and therefore the actual final surface temperatures attained are function of several parameters such as actual heat input (i.e heat generated) and the rate of heat dissipation. Sudden applications of load will give rise to setup of steep temperature gradients and surface temperature may rise above 950° C and at times high enough to cause surface melting. The body of the drum is relatively cool which may quench the heated surface on release of load. Thus, such sudden heating and cooling cycles involved, build of surface temperatures, and temperature gradients will lead to thermal cracking. Further, there can be machanical damage if the strength of the material is not enough and wearing and scoring may occur if the wear resistance in dry sliding condition is not adequate. Therefore, the gray iron for break drum should have good strength and resistance to failure by thermal cracking, growth and dry sliding wear. A gray iron with a minimum total carbon of 3.4%, a minimum CE of 4.0 and minimum tensile strength of about 30 kg/mm^2 will possess the above required characteristics.

The successive firings in an internal combustion engine setup fast temperature pulses on the flame face of the cylinder head. Each temperature cycle is followed by a cooling cycle and thus heating and cooling cycles are setup. The temperature rise in valve bridge may be above 350° C and the steep temperature gradients may setup. These conditions increase the risk of thermal cracking by build up of residual stresses as well as growth by dissociation. A low-alloy high duty gray iron having a T.S. of above 30 kg/mm^2 may be most resistant to thermal stress failure in cylinder heads. This is possible by good combination of fatigue strength, creep strength and thermal conductivity of such a material. A minimum of 3.2%C is desired in such iron.

There are other types of cast irons also recommended for the brake drums and cylinder heads. S.G. iron has superior machanical properties, better thermal shock resistance combined with good wear resistance and thus may prove to be a better choice than gray iron. However, its lower thermal conductivity is the main limitation which increases the risk of thermal cracking. Nevertheless, S.G. iron brake drums have proved very successful for the most severe service conditions involving violent braking under conditions of heavy load. By virtue of its relatively higher thermal conductivity, a pearlitic malleable iron will be slightly better than a pearlitic S.G. iron and is used for brake drums in certain cases.

10.3.3 Crankshafts and Gears

The principal meterial characteristics required for such applications are tensile strength, fatigue strength and wear resistance under high load, particularly for the gears. Table 10.1 gives machanical properties of importance for crankshaft applications of some materials commonly used.[76] It is well known that in general, bearing properties of all types of cast irons are superior to those of commonly used steel and therefore it is the fatigue properties that require to be compared of these two materials. It may be seen that the flake graphite high-duty irons do not have a fatigue strength comparable to steel, while the fatigue strength of the normalized S.G. iron having a minimum tensile strength of 80 kg/mm^2 will be fully comparable to forged steel having tensile strength of about 70 kg/mm^2. Its actual working fatigue strength will in fact be superior by virtue of its lower notch-sensitivity. Hence, the high strength grades of S.G. irons can safely subtitute forged steel having a tensile strength upto 70 kg/mm^2 for crank shaft applications. The higher percentage of elongation of such steels is not necessarily an advantage for such application from the functional points of view. S.G. irons besides having adequate properties for crank shaft applications also offer cost advantage as composed to steel. Moreover, S.G. cast iron crank shafts can be used either in the normalized or hardened and tempered conditions having a hardness of about 275-300 BHN without the need for a surface hardening treatment.

For gear applications, besides a high tensile strength and good fatigue properties, a high level of hardness is also required to resist high local pressures. Table 10.2 provides comparative picture of the important properties of the several materials commonly used for this purpose. It may be seen that some grades of S.G. irons have all the required properties comparable to those of plain or alloy steels. These grades of irons also have satisfactory level of hardness and excellent running-in properties and thus meet the essential requirements of the highly stressed gears. S.G.irons having a minimum tensile strength of 70 to 80 kg/mm^2 will be generally satisfactory for many such applications without requiring any surface-hardening treatment.

10.3.4 Pump Impellers and Marine Propellers

The above equipments are subjected to erosion by high velocities and severe turbulence in service and their combined action accelerates the overall rate of corrosion. Both the galvanic and selective corrosion occur. The requirements of propeller material vary depending on the size of the propeller and the type of the vessel to which it is to be fitted. However, for use of such propellers of large size in sea water even costly material like aluminum bronzes having high strength and corrosion resistance are recommended. For smaller propellers like those used in offshore fishing vessels, harbour craft, etc it is common to use manganese bronze and also sometimes gray iron. But both undergo selective corrosion like dezincification and graphitization, respectively in sea water. As such, an austenitic iron containing 21 to 24 % Ni and spheroidal graphite having good toughness (~20% elongation) will be suitable as it will be free from selective corrosion and will also with stand machanical damage as well as permit damaged blades to be straightened. The use of such iron for smaller size propellers is steadily growing.

TABLE 10.1: SOME TYPICAL PROPERTIES OF SOME CRANKSHAFT MATERIALS[76]

	Forged, carbon steel, quenched and tempered	*Forged Ni-Cr-Mo alloy steel, heat-treated*	*High duty cast iron*	*Acicular cast iron*	*High strength grades of S.G. Iron*			
					60/2	*70/2*	*80/2*	*90/2*
Tensile strength kg/mm^2	57	91	33	41	60	70	80	90
Yield strength or 0.2% proof stress, kg/mm^2	32	79	–	–	40	45	48	65
Elongation, %	25	23	<1	<1	2	2	2	2
Hardness, B.H.N.	160	269	220	280	210-280	230-300	260-330	270-340
Izod notched impact value, kg/cm^2	5	10	<0.2	0.25	<0.5	<0.5	<0.5	<0.5
Endurance limit. un-notched, kg/mm^2	24.9	45.7	11.3	18.9	25.5	28.0	32.0	34.0
Endurance limit, notched, kg/mm^2	12.6	27.6	9.4	14.21	15.3	16.8	18.8	19.8
Notch Sensitivity factor	1.98	1.66	1.20	1.33	1.67	1.67	1.70	1.72
Modulus of elasticity, $Ib/in^2 \times 10^{-6}$	29	29.5	18.21	22	25	25.5	25.5	25.5
Modulus of rigidity, Ib/ $In^2 X 10^{-6}$	11	11.65	8.6	8.6	9.75	9.95	9.95	9.95

TABLE 10.2: TYPICAL GEAR PROPERTIES OF SOME COMMONLY USED MATERIALS[76]

Sl No.	Materials	Tensile strength tons/in²	Tensile strength kg/mm²	Elastic modulus E ×10⁶ lbs/in²	Elastic modulus E × 10³ kg/mm²	Hardness BHN	Surface stress factor, lbs/in²	Surface stress Sc kg/mm²	Bending stress, Sb, lbs/in²	Bending stress, Sb, kg/mm²
1.	Cast iron (as cast)	12	18.9	12-16	8.4-11.3	165	1,025	0.72	5,800	4.08
2.	Cast iron(as cast)	16	25.2	15-18	10.5-12.7	210	1,350	0.95	7,600	5.34
3.	Cast iron (as cast)	22	34.6	18-22	12.7-15.5	220	1,450	1.02	10,500	7.38
4.	Alloyed iron	20	31.5	18-22	12.7-15.5	240-280	1,750	1.23	10,000	7.03
5.	Cast iron, high strength	22	34.6	18-22	12.7-15.5	300	2,100	1.48	10,500	7.38
6.	Malleable iron	20	31.5	24-27	16.9-19.0	140	850	0.60	12,000	8.44
7.	S.G. iron pearlitic/ ferritic	40-48	63-75.6	23-26	16.2-18.3	240	1,500	1.05	19000	13.36
8.	S.G. iron, hardened and tempered	60-70	94.5-110.2	23-26	16.2-18.3	340	2,500	1.76	30,000	21.09
9.	0.4% carbon steel, normalized	35	55.0	30	21.1	145	1,400	0.98	19,000	13.36
10.	0.5% carbon steel, surface hardened	35	55.0	30	21.1	160-550	2,800	1.97	17,000	11.95
11.	0.15% carbon steel, casehardened	32	50.4	30	21.1	750(DPN)	9,200	6.47	40,000	28.12
12.	5% nickel steel, casehardened	65	102.4	30	21.1	710(DPN)	12,000	8.44	50,000	35.15
13.	Phosphor bronze, sand-cast (BS:421)	12	18.9	16	11.3	69	700	0.49	7,000	4.92
14.	Phosphor bronze, chill-cast(BS:421)	15	23.6	16	11.3	82	850	0.60	8,500	5.98
15.	Phosphor bronze, centrifugally cast	17	26.8	16	11.3	90	1,000	0.70	10,000	7.03

As regards an impeller, it is subjected more to the effect of velocity and turbulence and its life will be lower than the casting. The type of the seawater or certain other type of water will also lead to graphitic corrosion if general cast iron is used. Therefore, even for such impeller, an austenitic cast iron impeller will minimize damage from all kinds of corrosion. However, another important cause of impeller failure is cavitation. A high hardness and high corrosion resistance are necessary to resist such cavitation. As such, a high-chromium type austenitic iron containing 13 to 18%Ni and 2.0 to 3.5% Cr will solve all such problems and will be superior to gray cast iron.

10.3.5 Wear Resistant Castings of Thermal Power Plants

Thermal power installations are one of the major sources of electric power generation. Depending on various operative conditions existing in boiler plants, castings are selected to meet specific requirements including the case of maintenance and cost of the equipment. In the above plants, castings of wear resisting type play a very important role. They are required to handle coal, ash and slurries. These castings in general are subjected to severe condition of abrasive wear. These castings are white in structure and are not machinable. The hardness may range from 300 to 500 HB. The service conditions besides hardness also require ductility and toughness for their satisfactory performance. A high compression strength together with an excellent resistance to deformation is also necessary. A variety of alloy cast irons are in use such as Cr-Mn , Cr-Mn-Ni, Ni-Cr-Mo and Cr-Mn-Ni-Mo alloy types[77-79] as given in Table 10.3. Of these, Ni-Hard type alloyed white cast iron is quite popular and is required in high tonnage in power plants. Its wear resisting properties are due to dense, hard graphite-free structure obtained with Cr and Ni additions. The typical applications are grinding rings, liners for P.F. mills and ash pump castings.

10.3.6 Machine Tool Components

A good machine tool is expected to finish a work piece in the minimum possible time, to specific dimensional accuracy with a super finish. Nowadays, machine tools have been developed utilizing full cutting capacity with spindle speeds of over 3000RPM and having complete freedom from vibration and chatter. To meet the requirements of higher speeds and feeding rate, the main body of the machine tool has to be very rigid, rugged and tough with large damping capacity, wear resistance and oil retaining[80] to withstand abnormal stresses caused by cutting and dynamic loads in service and weight of the work piece. They have also to withstand the wearing of surface by moving slides under load without any tendency to distort or vibrate. In the light of the above prerequisites, cast iron has been found to be the most ideal material for machine tool ensuring good machinability, higher strength and hardness, excellent surface finish, higher rigidity and the most outstanding damping properties.

TABLE 10.3: COMPOSITION AND PROPERTIES OF CAST IRONS USED IN BOILER INDUSTRY[79]

Chemical Composition	*Un Alloyed White Iron*	*Low-Alloy White Iron*	*Martenstic White Iron (Ni-Hard)*	*High-Carbon High-Chromium White Iron*
TC %	3.3-3.6	2.5-2.8	2.8-3.5	2.6-3.0
Si %	0.4-0.6	0.8-1.2	0.2-0.8	1.0 max
S %	0.15	0.10	0.10	0.05 max
P %	0.10	0.10	0.10	0.10 max
Mn %	0.2-0.6	0.50	0.50	0.70 max
Ni %	–	–	3.4-4.5	–
Cr %	–	0.8-1.2	1.4-2.5	25.0-30.0
Tensile strength (T/sq. in)	16-18	18-20	18-24	50-60
Hardness HB	550-650	400-450	450-650	500-550

Table 10.4 provides recommended chemical compositions of various cast irons with machanical properties desired for different applications of major machine tool components.

10.4 CONCLUSIONS

It is obvious from above discussions that before an appropriate type of cast iron is chosen for a particular application, a number of factors related to the service requirements must be carefully considered. The various factors which should be considered may include, operating temperature, risk of thermal shock, type of wear, type of the stress, distortion under load, type of corrosion which the components must with stand and also the overall

TABLE 10.4: RECOMMENDED CHEMICAL COMPOSITIONS FOR MAJOR MACHINE TOOL COMPONENTS[80]

	Casting of bed and bed groups	*Casting of gear and gear groups*	*Casting of head stock and head stock groups*	*Ordinary Castings*
Total carbon	2.8-3.0%	3.2-3.5%	3.2-3.5%	3.3-3.6%
Combined carbon	0.70%	0.50%	0.35%	0.30%
Silicon	1.4%	1.6 - 1.8%	1.8 - 2.0%	2.0%and above
Manganese	0.62%	0.66%	0.65%	0.6%
Nickel	1.4%	1.0%	0.6%	—
Chromium	0.40%	0.20%	—	—
Molybdenum	0.40%	—	0.2%	—
Phosphorus	0.34%	0.39%	0.30%	0.40%
Sulphur	0.11%	0.12%	0.12%	0.12%
Tensile strength	40000 to 50000 psi	30000 to 40000psi	30000 to 40000 psi	25000 to 30000 psi
Transverse strength	3000 to 5000 Ib	3000 Ib	3000Ib	3000Ib
Hardness	220 to 235 V	210 V	205 V	180-195 V

economics and the design changes possible to get best combination of properties, etc. The decision to use a particular material also should not be final and should be reviewed periodically to take advantage of technological developments taking place and to allow for changed demands in performance requirements.

Common Defects of Iron Castings and their Remedies

11

11.1 INTRODUCTION

Production of some defective work in a sand casting practice is practically unavoidable in spite of stringent supervision and inspection. It is true that defect free casting is the desire of all and therefore, a clear understanding of the causes for the occurrence of the defects and adoption of the possible remedial measures can go a long way in the reduction or elimination of the defects in castings. Various kinds of flaws or imperfections in the castings are regarded as true defects only when they affect the appearance or the satisfactory functioning of the castings. In general, in an iron foundry practice, no great concern is shown so long as the percentage of scrap castings falls within a normally acceptable percentage limit adopted by the foundry. However, it is possible to reduce significantly such accepted limit or percentage of the scrap castings and thereby to avoid the costly and time consuming salvage operations by careful control of the factors contributing to it. It is no doubt that any approach to the elimination of the casting defects much be on an economic basis.

A casting defect may arise from a single clearly defined cause or more commonly may be the result of a combination of factors. The various factors which may cause a defective work may be the use of unsuitable raw materials and the equipment appliances, poor casting and pattern design, unsatisfactory moulding and casting practice and/or the wrong managerial policy covering the purchase of raw materials, accessories and setting of production procedures etc. Therefore, to fix the causes, a thorough investigation of all the contributing factors is required and then proper remedial measures can be adopted. There is quite a large number of iron casting defects but attempt in this chapter will be made to present a simplified picture of some common defects which are frequently encountered in various iron casting foundries dealing with. their general appearance, probable causes and recommendations for their elimination.

11.2 CLASSIFICATION OR TYPES OF DEFECTS

A logical classification of various types of iron casting defects is rather a difficult task because of a wide range of factors contributing to their origin. However, they have been grouped into different categories using different basis[81-85]. A simple and rough classification of these defects can be made based on their nature and/or source of appearance. As such, the defects can be grouped under the following four headings:

1. Gas Defects
2. Surface Defects
3. Moulding and Pouring Defects
4. Solidification and Cooling Defects

The appearance, probable causes and methods of correcting these defects are discussed in brief as follows.

11.3 GAS DEFECTS

These defects take the form of blow holes and gas holes, surface or subcutaneous pinholes or intergranular porosity, depending on the immediate cause. Gases are emitted during pouring of moulds. The free escape of these gases during solidification of molten metal will depend on a number of factors like duration for which the metal remains molten, the amount of gas generated, the ease with which the evolving gas can escape out, etc. Any or combination of these factors can lead to entrapment of the gases produced. The various sources of gases which can give rise to gas defects are: (*i*) dissolved gases in the molten iron such as H_2 and N_2; (*ii*) reaction gases such as CO formed by reaction between the carbon in molten iron and oxygen in intimate contact with it, and (*iii*) gases evolved by moulds and cores containing gas producing additives such as moisture, binders, coal dust, etc. Most common different forms of gas defects, their causes and remedies can be discussed in turn.

11.3.1 Blow Holes and Gas Holes

These are rounded cavities which may either be spherical, elongated or flattened. They vary in size as well as in colour and occur mainly at the top surface of the casting. Blow holes occur in localized patches whereas gas holes are distributed throughout the casting.

Causes: Presence of high content of moisture, carbonaceous and gas producing materials in sand mixture, poor permeability of the mould/core, presence of clay balls and foreign particles in sand, etc.

Remedies: They can be ascertained by analyzing the causes that lead to these defects.

11.3.2 Pin Holes

These are small, elongated, smooth walled gas holes which occur mostly below the surface of the casting (Fig. 11.1). They are generally observed after cleaning or machining.

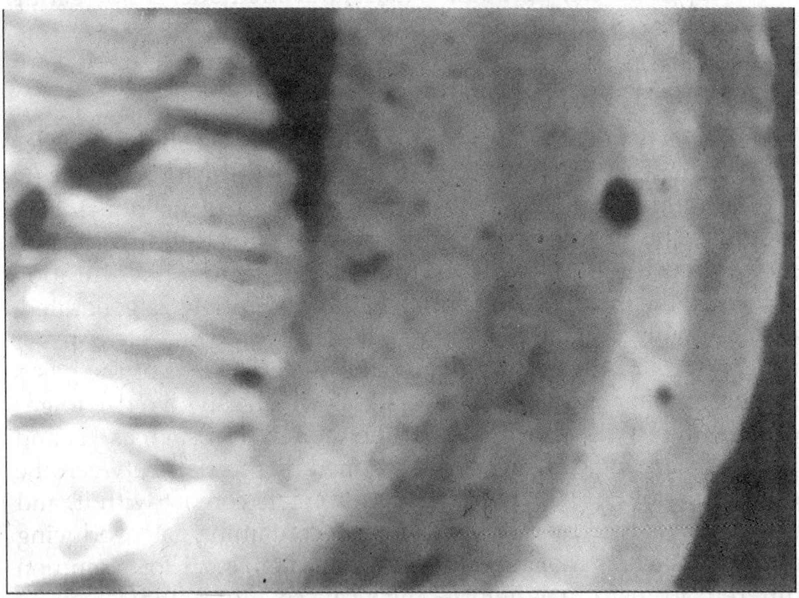

Fig. 11.1: Pin holes observed after machining the casting[85].

Causes: Hydrogen evolved during solidification of the casting is the main cause for the formation of the pin holes. The main source of hydrogen is water vapour, the decomposition of which in contact with molten iron liberates hydrogen in the atomic or nascent form which is readily soluble in iron. The sources of such water vapour are damp refractories, inadequately dried ladle linings and high moisture content of green sand mixtures. The presence of aluminium in iron accelerates the rate of reduction of water vapour, thus increasing the hydrogen availability for solution in iron. The sources of such aluminium are contaminated scrap metal and ladle inoculants.

Remedies: Elimination of all sources of moisture, use of well dried refractories and ladles, avoiding sources of addition of aluminium and increased use of coal dust.

11.4 SURFACE DEFECTS

This group of casting defects may include various kinds of surface irregularities such as surface roughness, sand adherence (metal penetration), several types of expansion defects like expansion scabs, buckles, rattails and erosion scabs.

11.4.1 Surface Roughness or Pebby Casting Surface

Casting surface not having required degree of smoothness for specific application.

Causes: Too coarse moulding sand, too high a pouring temperature of metal, high carbonaceous matter in the sand, too high or too low mixture in the sand, sand not properly rammed and uneven and incorrectly applied mould or core paints.

Remedies: Adopt corrective measures for the causes listed.

11.4.2 Expansion Scabs, Buckles and Rattails

Rough, irregular projection of the metal on the surface of the casting containing embedded sand (Fig. 11.2). Occur mainly on the top surface of the casting or in the areas of intense heating.

Causes: Highly superheated metal, slow pouring, uneven ramming, non-uniform expansion of sand.

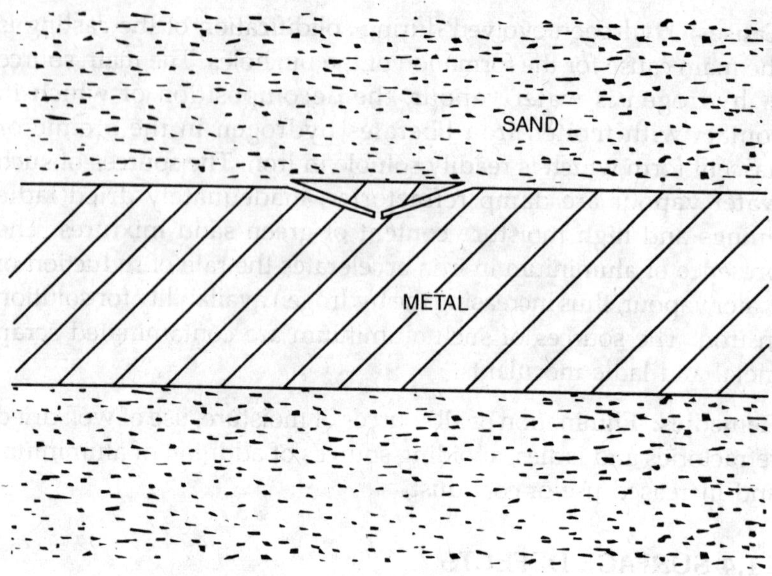

Fig. 11.2: Formation of expansion scab[82].

Mechanism of Formation: When molten metal flows into the mould cavity, its turbulence, shearing action, expansion of sand grains etc. try to tear off the surface of the mould. The expansion of the sand grains produces internal stresses too great for the rammed sand mass to withstand and leads to defects like scabs, buckles and rattails. Scab is the irregular projection of the metal on the surface of the casting. Rattail is an irregular line defect whereas buckle is a V-shaped indentation.

Remedies: Expansion of the sand face can be lowered by lowering the actual expansion of the sand or by lower heat input or by lowering the ramming density. The first step calls for the use of costly sands like zircon sand which can be justified in special cases. Lowering the heat input can be achieved by lowering the pouring temperature or by faster pouring. Lowering of ramming density can be a means to reduce overall expansion but such a step may be accompanied by swelling of the casting and the resulting unsoundness (due to mould wall movement). Another method may be to increase sand deformation to absorb sand expansion by additions of coal dust or pitch, wood flour and fibrous material. Coal dust increases sand deformation by softening at high temperature and making the sand plastic. Addition of wood four like material (at least 1%) acts as a cushion between the sand grains and thus allows expansion of the sand to be accommodated.

Thus, in general, use of other sands than silica such as olivine, zircon or calcined fire clay for preparing mould and mould wash, faster pouring and increasing hot deformation of sand by adding sufficient cushioning materials like wood flour, cereal binders, coal dust and pitch compounds, etc and fibrous materials like asbestous can be the possible remedies.

11.4.3 Erosion Scabs

Boiled or agitated molten metal which has partly eroded the sand leaving behind a solid mass of sand and metal at that particular spot.

Causes: High moisture and carbonaceous material leading to boiling of metal, improper mixing of sand ingredients and poor permeability, insufficient hot deformation and dry strength of the mould.

Remedies: Use of long and pliable fibrous material compared to short and stiff fibres and wood flour besides attending to the causes listed above.

11.4.4 Metal Penetration

It is also called as Burning-in and appears as a sand adherence produced on the casting surface when molten metal or the low melting constituent like fayalite fills the voids between the sand grains without displacing them.

Causes: localized over heating due to riser or gate location, oxidation of metal caused by gas aspiration and high pouring temperature, excessive pressure of metal during pouring.

Remedies: Use of sufficient carbonaceous and deoxidizing materials besides the measures to check the causes leading to this defect.

11.5 MOULDING AND POURING DEFECTS

The examples of such defects are crush, drops, shifts, swells, fins, misruns, cold shuts, etc.

11.5.1 Crush

It occurs due to displacement of sand at mould joints or core prints leading to production of irregular shaped cavities or projections on the casting.

Causes: Badly made mould joints causing uneven and excessive pressure on sand face, too heavy or uneven weighting, careless closing, cores too tight to place in core prints, etc.

Remedies: As obvious from above causes.

11.5.2 Drops

It is caused due to sand dropping from the top part of the mould or other hanging sections.

Causes: Too weak sand, non-uniform ramming and patched moulds, worn or in sufficient taper in the pattern or any sort of vibration in the mould.

Remedies: As obvious from above causes.

11.5.3 Swells

It is a gross imperfection in the casting dimensions than the permitted tolerance. It shows an enlarged casting section related to mould wall movement.

Causes: Soft ramming, excessive moisture, poor flowability of the sand, high pouring temperature and metallostatic pressure.

Remedies: High compaction of the sand and better flowability of the sand used.

11.5.4 Shifts

It is mismatch at the parting line of the casting (Fig. 11.3) from the specified dimensions due to misalignment or wrong positioning of the core.

Causes: Misaligned patterns in cope and drag, improper clamping, inadequate core print.

Remedies: A regular checking of the box pins, bushes, pattern fitting, etc.

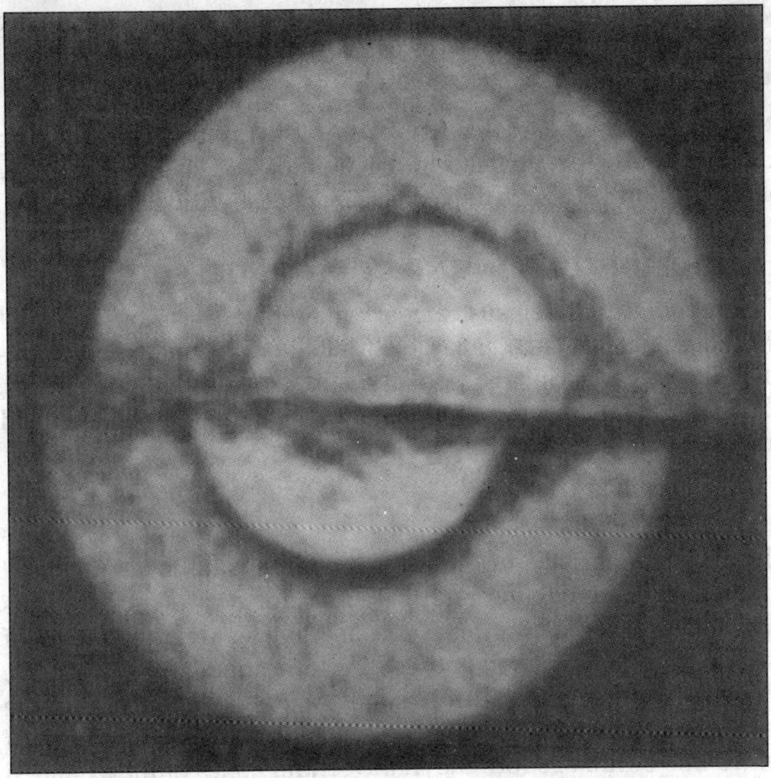

Fig. 11.3: Shift at the parting line of the casting[85].

11.5.5 Fins

Flattened excess metal coming out along the parting line of the mould or core.

Causes: Improper clamping of mould boxes, mould not properly vented.

Remedies: The corrective measures for the causes listed above.

11.5.6 Mis Runs and Cold Shuts

A misrun is a short run casting which lacks completeness due to failure of the metal to fill the mould cavity. A cold shut is produced when two streams of metal flowing from different regions in the casting meet without union. Cold lapping is a less severe form of the cold shut.

Causes: Insufficient fluidity of the metal, low pouring temperature, improper sizes of gating components, too thin metal section and too high moisture and volatile matter in the sand.

Remedies: Increase fluidity either by raising the pouring temperature or by preheating the mould, increase permeability of sand mixture and use the correct sizes of the gating components.

11.6 SOLIDIFICATION AND COOLING DEFECTS

Casting defects under this category may include various kinds of shrinkage defects such as large shrinkage cavity or pipe, centre-line shrinkage, shrinkage porosity, surface sinks and punctures, hard spot areas, inverse chill, kish graphite holes, hot tears, cold cracks, warpage, etc.

11.6.1 Shrinkage Defects

These defects arise from failure to compensate for liquid and solidification contraction and the actual form of defect depends upon a number of factors such as casting design, mode of solidification of the alloy and cooling condition. It may take the shape of large primary shrinkage cavity or pipe occurring in the heavy and isolated sections, secondary shrinkage in the form of centre-line-shrinkage forming in the central zones of the extended parallel walled sections. The long freezing range alloys show scattered shrinkage porosity whereas the skin forming short-freezing range alloys show surface sinks and punctures.

Causes: Lack of sufficient feed metal, heavy isolated sections, mould dilation due to soft ramming, use of too high a phosphorus content or too low a carbon equivalent of the iron composition and too high a pouring temperature.

Remedies: Use of proper casting design and feeder design, use of devices promoting directional solidification such as use of chills and insulating pads, use of correct composition of the iron and avoiding soft ramming.

11.6.2 Hard Spots (Hard Areas)

These are localized zones of very high hardness resulting from the formation of while iron structures in gray and ductile irons.

Causes: Wrong composition of the iron with respect to the section thickness used, thin sections of casting, gassy and cold metals, incorrect chill size used etc.

Remedies: Use of correct iron composition and inoculation, use of insulation of thin sections.

11.6.3 Inverse Chill

It is a condition in a gray, ductile or malleable iron casting section where the interior is chilled or white and the outer sections are gray or mottled.

Causes: Excess gas formation from a wet sand or core causing agitation of metal and upsetting in chemistry, presence of strong carbide stabilizer elements like Ti, S, etc., high pouring temperature.

Remedies: Reduce sulphur and avoid other carbide stabilizing elements, avoid high pouring temperature and use proper inoculation of the melt, avoid sources of hydrogen and other gases entering the metal.

11.6.4 Kish Graphite Holes

Appearance of free graphite separated from the molten iron occurring in clusters on sides and upper surfaces of the castings which are removed during cleaning forming holes.

Causes: Too high carbon equivalent composition of iron, low temperature metal causing separation of graphite in the ladle during pouring, excessive use of graphitizers.

Remedies: As obvious from the causes listed.

11.6.5 Hot Tears

They are cracks formed by the metal pulling itself apart while cooling in the mould around or just immediately after solidification of the metal and are characterized by a very irregular and jagged appearance and exhibit oxidation and a colouration due to heat effect. They are often found in the area of changes in section.

Causes: Internal stresses developed from hindered contraction caused by mould or core resistance and differential cooling of casting parts due to poor casting design, high pouring temperature, etc.

Remedies: Avoid abrupt changes in casting sections, use chills at hot spots and develop proper temperature gradient in the casting.

11.6.6 Cold Cracks

They are continuous cracks formed on the surface of the casting and occur at much lower temperatures than hot tears.

Causes: High internal stresses set up due to differential cooling of various parts of the casting, mishandling during removal of gates and risers or during shake-out.

Remedies: Cool the casting slowly and uniformly and use the casting design so that all the parts cool uniformly.

11.6.7 Warpage

It is an undesirable deformation of the casting developed during or after solidification of gray and white irons.

Causes: Unequal cooling of the parts due to bad casting design.

Remedies: Use proper camber allowance.

11.7 CONCLUSIONS

Casting defects are usually unavoidable but there are means by which such defects can be minimized and percentage of scrap casting can be reduced. These defects occur because some steps in the process of manufacturing have not been properly controlled. There can be more than one cause for the occurrence of a particular defect and therefore through investigation of all contributing factors must be made and proper remedies can be suggested.

12

Welding of Cast Irons

12.1 INTRODUCTION

Welding of cast irons is carried out for (*i*) repair of broken or worn parts; (*ii*) salvaging of foundry defects such as shrinkage porosity or other types of holes and; (*iii*) addition of structural components, e.g. joining of two or more castings. Repair of defects in new iron castings represents the largest single application of welding of cast irons. Defects such as casting porosity, sand inclusions, misruns, and shifts are commonly repaired by welding. The welding of simple castings to form assemblies is sometimes more economical than casting a complex shape. Iron castings can be also welded to other wrought shapes of different alloys such as steels, nickel alloys, etc for certain applications.

The welding procedures adopted for joining iron castings are selected to suit the type of cast iron to be welded. This is because some of the cast irons are readily welded, while others require great care to produce a sound weldment. There are some cast irons which are considered to be non-weldable. Gray cast irons have poor weldability. S.G. cast iron being ductile is more readily welded than gray irons. Before the different methods of welding of cast irons are discussed, it is worthwhile to know the general difficulties encountered during welding of cast irons.

12.2 METALLURGY OF WELDING OF CAST IRONS

Cast irons include a variety of ferrous alloys covering a wide range of compositions, microstructures and properties. When cast iron is welded, the weld metal is exposed to very rapid cooling as compared to cooling rates encountered during normal metal casting. Consequently, the properties of the weld metal and the other portions of the welded part exposed to different elevated temperatures (the HAZ-heat affected zone) differ from the remainder of the joint (base metal). Figure 12.1 shows typically the different zones formed across a weld joint. The structure of the heat affected zone depends upon parent metal composition and initial structure, the temperature attained and the cooling rate prevailing within this zone. During welding different levels of temperatures upto melting point are encountered as shown in the temperature distribution curve. It is commcn to find a coarse grained structure immediately adjacent to the fusion or weld zone. The cooling rates encountered depend upon a number of factors such as relative rates of heat dissipation and heat input, relative masses of weld metal and parent metal (for example, small weld metal undergoes most rapid cooling) and the degrees of pre/heating and post/heating employed. In general, the main difficulties encountered during welding of cast irons are due to:[86, 87]

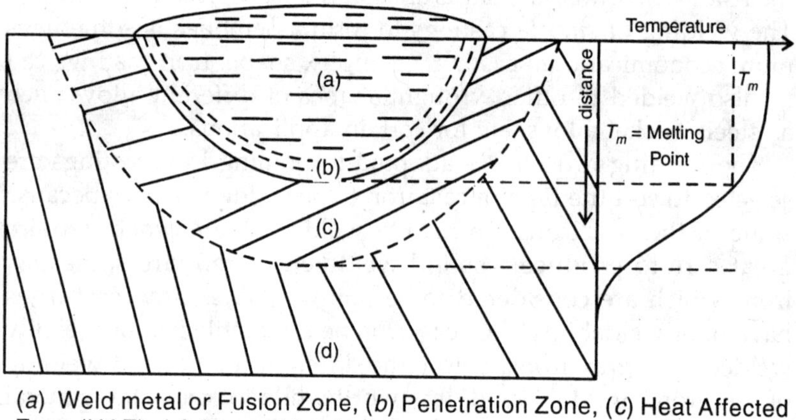

(*a*) Weld metal or Fusion Zone, (*b*) Penetration Zone, (*c*) Heat Affected Zone (HAZ), (*d*) Parent Metal

Fig. 12.1: Thermal conditions and structural zones formed across a weld zoint

1. **Formation of Hard or Unmachinable Weld Zone:** If the cast iron is rapidly cooled from the temperatures rear the melting point (as in fusion welding processes), carbon is retained in combined form (Fe_3C) and the welded zone becomes hard and unmachinable due to formation of iron

carbide. When steel filler rods are employed, hardness in weld metal zone may arise from diffusion of carbon from the parent metal to steel filler material with the formation of martensite. Therefore, if rapid cooling can be avoided, risk of getting hard weld zone will be reduced. When an isolated zone of a large casting is welded, heat is conducted away fast from the weld zone to cold metal surrounding it but this effect can be reduced by a preheating operation applied during welding which prevents a too steep temperature gradient set-up between the weld metal and the parent metal. Such preheating may be done with the help of a gas torch or for large casting using a charcoal furnace.

2. **Cracking, either in the Parent Metal (HAZ) or in Weld Metal:** During welding, thermal stresses are developed due to uneven heating and cooling of the weld and parent metal and consequent unequal expansion and contraction of these parts. In complex castings, particularly large stresses are set-up in colder portion of the casting due to uneven expansion and contraction. Under such circumstances, for a material like gray iron which lacks ductility, the cracking tendency will be severe. Further, cracking may also take place in weld metal portion due to formation of a highly brittle eutectic material if the iron contains more than 0.5% phosphorus, particularly during arc welding where conditions of thermal schock are severe. In general, application of preheating and/or postheating can assist in prevention of cracking by equalizing the rates of expansion and contraction in weld and parent metals.

3. **Formation of Unsound Weld Metal due to lack of adherance between Weld Deposit and Parent Metal:** The oxidation of metal during welding and also the welding of improperly prepared surfaces may give rise to lack of adherance between parent metal and the weld metal and thus may cause unsound weldment. The formation of ferrous oxide layer at the welding interface as well as formation of white iron due to loss of carbon and silicon due to oxidation taking place during welding may lead to such situation of bad adherance. The use of proper flux

may provide protections against such oxidation taking place during welding. Fluxes used are usually composed of borates or boric acid, soda ash and small amounts of other compounds such as sodium chloride, ammonium sulphate, and iron oxide

4. **Loss of Alloying Elements due to Oxidation and hence, a Change in Structure and Properties of the Weldment:** Besides creating problem of unadherance between weld deposit and the parent metal, the oxidation occurring during welding may also change the composition and thereby structure and properties of the weldment. The remedy is to use a proper flux or protective atmosphere during welding as guards against oxidation. Use of a proper flux performs several functions such as (*i*) it keeps weld metal surface clean; (*ii*) protects metal from oxidation during welding; (*iii*) dissolves oxides and other impurities; (*iv*) prevents loss of volatile elements present; and (*v*) improves fluidity of weld metal.

Hence, the above remedies as suggested can take care of many problems encountered during welding. The castings should also be slowly cooled after welding to reduce further the internal stresses developed. In some cases, a stress relieving heat treatment may be necessary.

12.3 PREPARATION FOR WELDING

It is a very important step for successful welding that the parts to be repaired by welding are properly prepared. The edges of the parts to be welded should be cleaned and prepared by chipping and grinding to form a single or double V grooves to ensure good metal penetration and fusion of the deposited metal. Double V grooves are used for thicker castings. A proper gap should be maintained at the root of the groove and the base angles of 60 to 120° are used as shown in Fig. 12.2. Base angles of 60-70° are generally required for virtually all of the filler metals and welding processes.[88]

When a defect is to be repaired by welding, it must be removed first by grinding, gouging or machining otherwise its presence will lead to poor weld quality. The area then should be properly inspected to ensure that the defect has been completely removed.

The size of the weld joint must be kept to a minimum to reduce stress levels resulting from uneven thermal contraction rates between weld metal and the base metal.

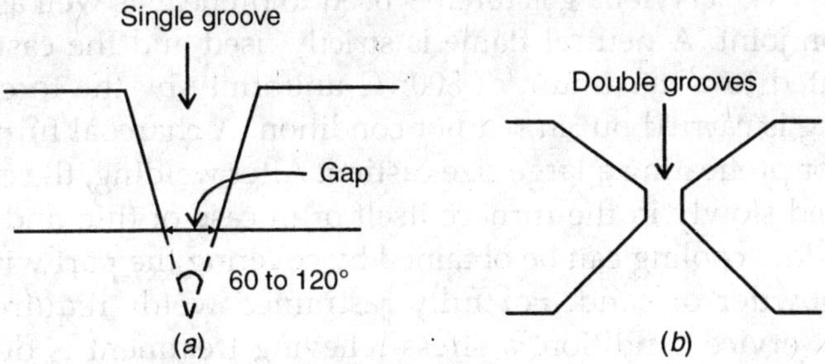

Fig. 12.2: Single and double grooves of weld joints

Before welding, the area to be welded should be thoroughly cleaned free of any dirt, grease or paint. Repeated degreasing with the help of a good solvent is necessary to ensure removal of such materials. Heating the casting to 350 to 500° C for 15 to 30 minutes further helps removal of oil and grease impregnated in the casting. The surface of the casting should preferably be also removed in the immediate area of the weld to ensure removal of such contaminants.

12.4 WELDING PROCESSES

The various welding processes used may be broadly divided into two major groups and their sub groups as follows.[86-88]

1. Fusion Welding Processes in which parts to be welded are melted.
2. Non-Fusion Welding Processes in which parts to be welded are not melted.

1. Fusion Welding Processes
   (i) Gas Welding
   (ii) Metal Arc Welding
   (iii) Thermit Welding
   (iv) Burning-On
2. Non-Fusion Welding Processes
   (i) Braze Welding or Brazing
   (ii) Powder Welding

12.4.1 Oxy-Acetylene Gas Welding

This welding process is widely used for welding of cast irons, but it requires massive heat inputs both for preheating and welding. A large oxy-acetylene gas torch is used to preheat as well as weld the iron joint. A neutral flame is strictly used and the casting is preheated to a maximum of 800° C uniformly by the torch and welding is carried out in red hot condition. A charcoal furnace is used for preheating a large size casting. After welding, the casting is cooled slowly in the furnace itself or in case of thin and small parts, slow cooling can be obtained by covering the part with dry lime powder or sand. For fully restrained welds required for severe service condition, a stress-relieving treatment is desired, immediately after welding. This consists of heating to 595 to 610° C for one hour per inch of the section thickness of the casting and then cooling at a rate of 10° C per hour or less until the weld has cooled at least to 370° C.

The filler metal used may be gray iron or other material in form of square or round bars of similar composition as parent metal. It is customary to use a high silicon (3.5% Si) iron filler rod to obtain a machinable weld deposit. Rods containing 1.25 to 1.75% Ni are also used where high quality weld is required. The flux is invariably used for the purpose as out lined earlier. The heat affected zone obtained by gas welding is larger than produced by more intense and localized electric arc welding and therefore tendency of the weldment to distort is greater in gas welding.

12.4.2 Metal-Arc or Shielded Metal-Arc Welding

These processes are used where it is necessary to weld the casting in cold condition or where heavy metal deposit in large casting is desired. A flux coated consumable electrode (Fig. 12.3) which provides the source of heat (arc) and also acts as filler metal is used. The gas and slag shielding are derived from the mineral coatings on the filler rod. The heat affected zone formed is small which minimizes the distortion. The electrode normally used in this method is a steel electrode which is fluxed coated. Stainless steel electrodes are also used. Besides these, electrodes based on Ni alloy such as Ni-Fe or Ni-Cu are also widely used for gray, malleable and S.G. iron castings. The parts to be welded may be preheated to lower superheat such as upto 300° C although cold welding processes is more common. A stress relieving treatment may be useful. Such arc welding processes have the advantages of a large selection of consumables, low-cost power supplies and all-position welding and therefore most widely used.

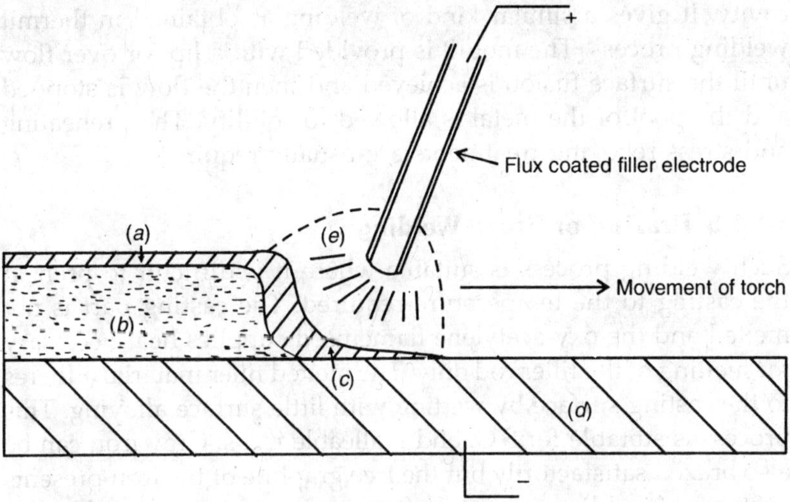

(a) Slag Shield, (b) Weld metal, (c) Weld pool, (d) Parent metal, (e) Gas shield

Fig. 12.3: Shielded metal-arc welding process.

12.4.3 Thermit Welding

It is a special welding process in which hot liquid metal for welding purpose is produced in a refractory lined vessel by a highly exothermic chemical reaction between iron oxide and aluminum powder as:

$$Fe_2O_3 + 2A1 \rightleftarrows A1_2O_3 + 2Fe + Heat$$

The above reaction may be some times explosive in nature besides generating a large amount of heat needed for melting and superheating iron. The necessary alloying elements are added in suitable forms to yield a hot metal of desired chemical composition. The hot metal is poured into a mould box specially prepared around the weld joint and good quality weld is attained. This process is used for weld repairing of heavy structures or sections such as machinery bases and frames and the welding process can be carried out at any place.

12.4.4 Burning-On

This is a simplified method of filling a large shrinkage cavity and pipes formed in the casting. The superheated metal for this is obtained from a cupola and the metal is allowed to flow continually over the cavity to be filled by building a sand mould around the cavity. It gives a similar kind of welding as obtained in thermit welding process. The mould is provided with a lip for over flow until the surface fusion is achieved and then the flow is stopped and the pool of the metal is allowed to solidify. The preheating and stress relieving treatments are usually required.

12.4.5 Brazing or Braze Welding

Such welding process is suitable where it is difficult to preheat the casting to the temperature required. The casting part is not melted and the oxy-acetylene flame used supplies heat necessary for melting of the filler rod only. The melted filler material adheres to the casting surface by wetting with little surface alloying. This process is suitable for S.G. and malleable irons. Gray iron can be also brazed satisfactorily but the free graphite of the iron presents problem of welding in joint surfaces and must be removed before brazing to get a good bond. The 60-40 brass or bronzes of suitable compositions are normally employed as filler materials. The preheating upto 400° C is desirable but not so essential as in fusion welding since lower temperatures are used. The stress reliving is not usually required and flux is used. However, the strength of the weld is much less than the parent metal.

12.4.6 Powder Welding

In this process, a finely divided metal powder is fed through a metering device into the oxygen stream of the oxy-acetylene flame. As the powder passes through the flame, it is preheated and melts as it reaches the surface of the base metal. The surface wetting and inter-diffusion occurs which develop the bond. Ni-base powder welding alloys melt between 950 to 1000° C and the base cast iron is preheated upto 200 to 350° C and reaches 700 to 800° C during application of the powder filler metal. However, melting does not occur. No flux is required. There is no carbide formation and rate of cooling of the weld is controlled by gas torch to prevent the formation of martensite. This process is used for gray, malleable and S.G. irons and alloy irons. The weld strength is similar to that of the parent metal. The residual stresses formed are much lower than fusion welding processes and the cost of the equipment is much lower than arc welding process.

12.5 WELDING OF DIFFERENT CAST IRONS

Specific details of the welding processes and meterials used for different types of cast irons are as follows. [89-98]

12.5.1 Welding of Gray Irons

Practically, all the welding processes, as discussed above are used for welding of gray cast irons depending upon the requirement of a defect to be repaired or the amount of the weld metal needed. Oxy Acetylene gas welding and Metal-Arc welding are the most commonly used processes. The gas welding is generally used for defect repair, but can also be used for production of assemblies. A high velocity gas torch that produces a concentrated flame pattern should be used. Gray iron weldments are succeptible to the formation of gas porosity. This can be taken care by slowing the cooling rate during weld formation so that the gas has sufficient time to escape from the weld pool. A minimum preheat of 205 to 315° C is recommended which reduces the cracking tendency and also helps in reducing the porosity. The most common arc welding electrodes for gray iron are nickel or nickel-iron alloys. A high-silicon gray iron rod is commonly used as filler metal for gas welding. A post weld stress relieving treatment is recommended, particularly for complex castings.

12.5.2 Welding of Malleable and White Irons

Superior tensile strength and ductility of malleable iron compared with that of gray iron makes this material more suitable for welding either for repairing or for joining two or more pieces together. However, the danger of carbide and martensite formation during the welding process is always there and care has to be taken to prevent or reduce these.

Beside gas welding, metal arc welding, brazing and powder welding processes are used for welding of malleable irons. Because most malleable iron castings are small, preheating is seldom used. However, for heavy section and highly restrained joints, preheating upto 150 to 200° C and post weld malleablizing annealing are recommended. If necessary, small castings can be stress relieved by heating up to 540° C. The ferritic malleable irons have the highest weldability of all other grades of malleable irons. The pearlitic grades of malleable irons have higher cracking susceptibility when welded because of higher combined carbon content.

Gas welding is often used for repair of small defects while the casting is in the white iron condition, before malleablizing. White iron welding rods are used similar to base metal composition. After welding, the casting is given its normal malleablizing heat treatment. Metal-arc welding with steel eletrodes is used in joining malleable iron. The braze welding, using a copper alloy welding rod is a good method of offering a relatively strong and machinable joint in malleable irons.

Chilled and white cast irons are abrasion resistant cast irons having cast structures free of graphitic carbon. Because of their high hardness and brittleness, they are generally considered unweldable.

12.5.3 Welding of S.G. Irons

Like malleable, S.G. cast irons can be more easily welded for their similar strength and ductility characteristics. In gas welding process, normally nodular iron filler rods containing higher than usual levels of Mg & Ce are used to offset losses during welding. The pre heating is usually not necessary due to high heat input of the gas welding process but a post weld heat treatment is necessary for maximum ductility. Normalizing or annealing treatments are employed.

In metal-arc or shielded metal-arc welding of S.G. iron casings, a 55% Ni-Fe electrode is often recommended since the strength and toughness of the weld metal obtained is comparable to that of the parent metal. It is generally necessary to pre heat the ferritic grade of S.G. iron to 120 to 180° C and the pearlitic grade to 200 to 300° C for avoiding cracking in the heat affected zone. A post weld heat treatment, full annealing for the ferritic grade and normalizing for the pearlitic grade is essential, if maximum mechanical properties are required from the heat affected zone.

Therefore, for obtaining maximum ductility, like malleable iron casting, the welded S.G. iron castings should be immediately transferred to a hot furnace for full annealing treatment and normal sequence of heating and cooling should be followed.

The powder welding process is also successfully used for S.G. iron castings as carbide formation is avoided and comparable weld strength is obtained. However, the braze welding is not recommended if original strength must be achieved since at least 20% strength reduction takes place as result of braze welding.

12.5.4 Welding of Alloy Cast Irons

Alloy cast irons are used in special applications which require good corrosion, heat, abrasion or wear resistance properties. It is essential that such properties are retained in the weldment after the welding. Welding is therefore generally not recommended to abrasion resistant cast irons as they have limited resistance to thermal shock. Welding is some times employed for repairing or attaching parts to other machine components. Gas welding is preferred over arc welding as former is not so prone to cause cracking. Arc welding is done with stainless electrodes if the welded area is not subjected to abrasion. In case abrasion resistance is required, the electrode used should produce weld metal of similar abrasion resistance as the base metal. The casting in all above cases is preheated from 315 to 480° C and slowly cooled after welding. Stress relieving at 205° C should be used.

13

Inspection and Testing of Iron Castings

13.1 INTRODUCTION

In iron foundries, quality control systems are designed to ensure that castings are produced with a certain level of quality that is acceptable to both the customer and the supplier. At various stages during the manufacturing and particularly on the finished castings, some inspection is required to see that the specifications of casting quality are being maintained. Castings with obvious visible defects are quickly rejected. However, castings which are dimensionally or metallurgically defective may require special measurements or tests before they are detected.

Inspection of iron castings normally consists of checking for shape and dimensions, coupled with aided and unaided visual inspection for external discontinuities and surface quality. Various kinds of tests performed for mechanical properties along with chemical analyses are supplemented by those of nondestructive inspection including leak testing and proof loading and all these are used to ensure the soundness of the castings. Since these various inspection procedures add to the cost of the product, a prior consideration is required to determine the amount of the inspection needed to maintain adequate control over the quality required. In some cases, full inspection of each individual casting may be required where as in other cases, sampling procedures may be sufficient to maintain the quality of the casting.

13.2 TYPES OF INSPECTION

The inspection procedures adopted for quality testing of castings may be classified as follows.[99-106]

1. Visual Inspection
2. Dimensional Inspection
3. Metallurgical Inspection

13.2.1 Visual Inspection

This is adopted to check the surface quality and obvious surface defects of the casting such as cracks, tears, blow holes, scabs, metal penetration, swells, etc. which are immediately detected by visual examination of the casting. It can be done by naked eye or sometimes aided by magnifying lense or low power microscope. Surface quality of the casting is also judged by chemical etching, liquid penetrant inspection, eddy current inspection and magnetic particle inspection which can also reveal discontinuities situated immediately below the surface.

13.2.2 Dimensional Inspection

This is adopted to check the dimensional accuracy of the cast products and involves the principles of gauging as it is applied to any machine element. These dimensional checks are made with the manual micro meters as well as manual and automatic gauges. Various types of gauges such as height and depth gauges, contour gauges, snap and plug gauges, etc. can be applied to the castings. The latter can be also sectioned to check metal wall thickness.

13.2.3 Metallurgical Inspection

It includes chemical analysis, mechanical property tests, evaluation of casting soundness and product testing of special properties (physical tests) such as corrosion resistance, wear resistance and antifriction properties, response to heat treatment, strength in assemblies, conditions of surface coatings and surface treatments and others. The chemical analysis is performed to determine whether the composition is within allowable limits or not. The carbon equivalent measurement or other direct methods give an indication of chemical compositions. Castings and test bars are tested to see that mechanical property specifications are met for which tensile, hardness, transverse strength, impact resistance, fatigue and other property are tested in accordance with standard procedures adopted.

The various kinds of casting defects like shrinkage cavities, gasholes, general porosity, hot tears, cracks, entrained slag and sand inclusions, etc. are all considered as contributing to lackness of the casting soundness when they are present. Various kinds of non-destructive testing methods used for detecting internal discontinuities are radiographic, ultrasonic and eddy current inspection.

Besides inspection procedures adopted at various stages of the casting manufacture to guide for the corrective measures to be adopted, some form of final inspection is inevitably used even if this is only on a sample of the batch of castings. Frequently, this final inspection involves some form of non-destructive testing and if the final inspection is to be carried out on 100 percent of the castings, then a non-destructive testing applied to iron castings are different when applied to final inspection than when applied to proto-type castings and further different requirements are necessary if the castings to be inspected are large or small. For example, for the final inspection of large numbers of small castings, the inspection technique must be rapid, easy to operate and cheap and only as accurate as is required by the quality standard acceptable. However, for the examination of large castings, speed is not so essential and since these castings will have a higher inherent value, a greater accuracy from the testing is required. This will certainly lead to increase in the testing costs.

13.3 METHODS OF INSPECTION AND TESTING

Inspection of castings is generally limited to visual and dimensional inspections, weight testing and hardness testing However, to check the complete quality, additional methods of non-destructive inspection are usually adopted. The first visual inspection operation is usually performed immediately after shakeout of the casting. This ensures that the major obvious defects or imperfections are detected at the earliest possible to permit early corrective action to be taken with a minimum of the scrap loss. Many intricately cored castings are extremely difficult to measure accurately, particularly their internal sections. In order to ensure that their sections are correct in thickness, the first indication about the discrepancies can be obtained by accurately weighing each casting. There should be no additional weight that would make the finished product heavier than permissible. The various methods of inspection and testing adopted for detecting casting defects and properties can be broadly grouped into following categories:

1. Methods for Detection of Surface Defects
2. Methods for Detection of Internal Defects
3. Methods for Measurement of Properties.

13.3.1 Detection of Surface Defects

All the methods in this category require clean and relatively smooth surfaces of the casting for effective results of examination.

13.3.1.1 Visual Examination

This is most important test adopted for iron castings which is closely followed by measurement of vital dimensions. Various kinds of aids to such inspection are adopted which include adequate illumination of the areas under inspection and use of necessary gigs and fixtures for checking measurement. Such visual inspection will be able to eliminate castings with major surface imperfections such as misruns, cross-joints and blowholes. The areas of the castings from where risers have been removed should be carefully examined for presence of any defect.

13.3.1.2 Magnetic Crack Detection or Magnetic-Particle Inspection

This method is frequently used in iron foundries to detect presence of smaller cracks on the surface or slightly sub-surface defects which may not be detected by visual examination. In this technique, a magnetic field is set-up in the casting or in the part of the casting being examined either by passing a heavy electric current through the casting or immersing the casting in the magnetic field set-up by a coil carrying electric current or by a permanent magnet. If any crack is present in the casting and interrupt the magnetic field in the casting, there will be a magnetic flux leakage at the position of the crack and this leakage will be defected by magnetic particles applied as a dry powder or in a suspension in a liquid applied as magnetic ink. For best sensitivity, the magnetic particles are covered during manufacture to form a proprietary fluorescent magnetic ink and the casting is viewed under an ultraviolet light.

In such conditions, areas where the magnetic particles have accumulated, as being associated with the cracks present, stand out brightly against the dark back ground. A difficulty inherent in this technique is that the crack detection efficiency varies with the orientation of the crack because a crack which runs in the same direction as the magnetic field will not interrupt with the magnetic field and therefore can not be detected. Normally, two separate tests in almost perpendicular directions should be carried out to detect the presence of the crack.

The magnetic crack detection technique is widely used on both the small as well as large castings. Small castings are completely magnetized during the test but in case of lage castings only small areas of the casting are magnetized by passing a current through this localized area.

13.3.2 Detection of Internal Defects

The magnetic particle method does not indicate the depth of the crack and is therefore restricted to the detection of the surface or subsurface defects. For detection of internal defects either ultrasonic testing or radiographic examination can be used. Both of these tests are slow in operation and require skilled workers to operate. They are normally used for inspection of large castings or inspection of prototype castings, although some times used for the 100 percent inspection of small castings as well.

13.3.2.1 Ultrasonic Testing

It is a non-destructive testing method in which beams of high-frequency acoustic energy are introduced into the casting to detect the internal defects like cracks, inclusions and internal ruptures and to measure the thickness of the material or the distance at which flaw exists. When ultrasonic beams are introduced at one casting surface, they will be reflected from the opposite surface of the casting after a suitable time interval. Internal Defects will also reflect the sound waves but the time required for the reflection will be less than that of the opposite casting surface. The interfaces and defects thus interrupt the beam and reflect a portion of the incident acoustic energy. The amount of the energy reflected is a function of the nature and orientation of the defect or interface as well as the acoustic impedance of such a reflector. The energy which is reflected from various interfaces or defects is used to define the presence and location of the defects, the thickness of the material or the depth of a defect beneath the casting surface.

The efficiency of this method of inspection of iron castings is governed by the ultrasonic properties of the material it self as well as the intricacies of the shape of the casting. Cast irons and especially gray irons scatter ultrasonic energy more than other materials commonly examined by this method such as steels and aluminum alloys. This scatter reduces the resolution of the defect and makes interpretation of the ultrasonic indications more difficult. It is therefore necessary that comparatively low ultrasonic frequencies be used for satisfactory energy penetration. In S. G. irons and high grade gray irons, the ultrasonic frequency commonly used is 2.5 MHz, but in low grade gray irons having a coarser graphite structure, it may be necessary to reduce the frequency of the ultrasonic energy for the test to about, 1 MHz. The use of such frequencies limits the smallest size of the defect that can be detected.

The major problems which arise in the use of ultrasonic testing of cast irons are those which are caused by the intricacy of the shape of the casting and also by their surface conditions. However, for efficient ultrasonic testing, it is necessary to maintain intimate contact between the ultrasonic probe system and the casting under test. Since this is difficult to maintain such contact with the rough surface, it is common to use a grease as a coupling material which to some extent, alleviates this problem. However, if the casting surface is curved and the probe surface is flat, good coupling between the two can be maintained over a small area with a consequent reduction in the efficiency of this test. Further, the castings frequently have back surfaces which are not parallel to the front surface and hence, the ultrasonic pulse energy that is transmitted to the casting does not reflect back into the receiver to establish a back wall echo on the ultrasonic test set. The presence of back wall echo is very helpful to the ultrasonic operator since it enables him to ensure that adequate coupling has been achieved between the probe and the casting.

The ultrasonic testing method can be very useful for detecting internal defects in gray iron and S.G. iron casting sections of 1/2 to 6 inches and can be also used for measuring wall thicknesses.

This second facility is useful when the casting wall thickness can not be measured by other mechanical means and the core shift also can be readily detected. For getting accurate measurement of the casting wall thickness, the instrument used needs prior calibration.

13.3.2.2 *Radiographic Examination*

Radiographic examination is a method which uses X-rays or gamma radiations to examine the interior of the castings. It is a process of testing castings using penetrating radiations of X-rays or γ-rays and an imaging medium such as X-ray film or an electronic device. In passing through the material, some of the radiation is attenuated, while the radiation that passes through the material forms an image. This radiographic image is generated by variations in the intensity of the emerging beam. The internal flaws present in the cast product such as gas entrapment or nonmetallic inclusions create variations in casting material thickness resulting in localized dark or light spots on the image. Such a radiographic process produces a permanent image on a film. It is also possible to view such image on a fluorescent screen or image intensifier.

X-ray tubes are used for the production of X-rays and γ-rays are obtained from a radioactive source like a radium capsule or a cabalt-60 capsule or other source and they are shorter in wave lengths than X-rays but have more penetrating power. The distance from the X-rays or γ-rays source to the casting, its section thickness, exposure time and many other details must be properly selected to give satisfactory results. Since most defects transmit the short-wave length light better than the sound metal does, the X-ray film is darkened more where the defects are in the line of the X-ray beam. Thus, radio-graphic examination gives a permanent film record of the defect that is easy to interpret and has established standards. In fact, it is one of the oldest and the most widely used non-destructing tests of iron castings. Of course, this method is expensive and therefore is only used when justified.

The choice of use of X-radiography or gamma radiography depends on the technical requirements and on the equipment available. In general, X-radiography gives better results on iron castings of section thickness upto about one inch and gamma radiography is preferable on thick sections of 4 to 12 inches. In the intermediate range of thicknesses, both X-ray and γ-ray can give acceptable results. X-rays are more intense than the γ-rays obtained from the covenient size of isotope sources, and hence, the exposures for X-rays are generally less than the γ-rays for which exposure required may be of many hours duration.

Difficulties arise in radiography of small castings which are caused by the shape of the casting and by the number of changes in cross-sectional area that are inherent in many designs of the castings. All these factors require a skilled operator to use such tests and interpret the results. Under good conditions, radiography can detect defects equivalent to about 2 percent of the section thickness. However, it is not possible except by specialized techniques to determine exactly the location of the defect in the casting section. A relatively recent development in radiographic techniques is the advent of fluoroscopic image intensifying systems which may make radiography to be more suitable for the routine examination of many castings. In these techniques, the radiations transmitted through the casting are allowed to fall on a fluoroscopic screen and the image formed on that screen is amplified by the image intensifier and the electronic systems. Such a technique allows rapid examination to be made, but requires rather elaborate and expensive equipment.

13.3.3 Measurement of Properties

A casting may be rejected either because of unacceptable presence of casting defects or due to bad material properties. This is because a casting which is too weak is just as defective and will fail in service just as quickly as a casting which contains large internal cavities or surface cracks. This necessitates that for accepting a casting there should be also ways to assess its properties to meet required specifications which may be desirable in service for its satisfactory performance. There are therefore methods available for measurement of properties of cast products many of which are non-destructive in nature.

In cast irons, there are two important parameters which govern the properties of iron castings viz. the shape and distribution of the graphite and the matrix structure. For example, irons containing spherical graphite and/or those having pearlitic matrix are stronger than those containing flake graphite and/or having ferritic matrix. It is thus necessary to check both of these two parameters by some tests in order to ensure that iron castings are within the specified limits of characteristics. The tests available for characterizing these parameters are non-destructive types as discussed below.

13.3.3.1 Sonic Testing

This technique is used for assessment of the graphite form of iron castings. In this test, the resonant frequency of the casting is determined. This characteristics is governed by the elastic modulli and since the latter vary with the form of the graphite, a correlation can be determined between the resonant frequency and the form of the graphite. Castings containing spherical shape of the graphite have a higher resonant frequency than the same design of the casting with flake graphite. This test thus enables a quick detection of the graphite form which can be interpreted in terms of the tensile strength of the casting material. It is necessary to establish a correlation curve for each separate design of the casting to be tested and therefore, the sonic testing is most suitable when large numbers of the same design of the casting are to be tested. Hence, this method is not applicable to small quantities of the castings and in general, not applicable to large castings.

13.3.3.2 Eddy Current Testing

This test is designed to assess the matrix structure of the iron castings and relies for its operation of the variation of the magnetic properties of the ferritic and pearlitic matrix structures. Ferrite has high magnetic permeability whereas pearlite has a low magnetic permeability and thus, a measurement of the magnetic permeability of the casting gives an indirect assessment of the amount of the ferrite or pearlite present in the structure.

This test is normally performed on a comparative basis in which these magnetic properties of the casting under test are compared with those of a reference casting. Any differences between the magnetic properties can be displayed on an electronic unit and can be used to separate those castings with the same magnetic properties from those with different properties. However, the eddy current technique is again limited to one design of the casting and needs separate calibrations for different designs of the castings. As such this technique is most suitable for the inspection of large numbers of the same design of the casting.

13.3.3.3 Mechanical Property Testing

As mentioned earlier, in addition to chemical analysis, castings are also tested to see that all mechanical property specifications are closely met. There are standard procedures and test pieces specified for testing of properties like tensile strength, hardness, transverse, impact and fatigue strengths and other relevant properties which are followed to ensure that castings meet these property requirements as laid down in their specifications.

Hardness testing is generally used to check the effectiveness of the heat treatment given to the casting. Its correlation with the tensile strength enables a rough predication of the tensile strengths of the cast products. The Brinell hardness test is most frequently used. However, this test is unsuitable for measuring higher levels of hardness (above 600 H B), for which either the Rockwell or the Vickers hardness test is performed,

13.3.3.4 Pressure Testing

This test, in addition to locating leaks in the casting, is performed on gray iron spun pipe castings to check the overall strength of the casting (proof loading) in resistance to bursting under hydraulic pressure. The equipments are available for sealing off such casting and finding the leaks. The proof loading by hydraulic pressure involves introducing a fluid, oil or water into the casting. The casting is then subjected to a pressure which is in excess of the maximum stress the casting is supposed to in-counter in service.

13.4 CONCLUSIONS

Hence, a large number of inspection methods are available to control the quality and specifications of iron castings within specified limits. New developments are takings place in inspection methods to meet the production demands and some of them are fully automated. For examples, various installations are already in operation with automated magnetic crack detection, automated sonic and eddy current testing. However, such automated test systems can only be applied to long run of castings of the same pattern to justify the high costs associated with the use of expensive equipments necessary for the mechanical handling of the castings and for the sorting of the castings after inspection.

14

Design of Iron Castings

14.1 INTRODUCTION

Casting design is a very important aspect of the manufacture of a casting as any mistake committed at the design stage not only will increase the cost of the manufacture but is also responsible for production of defective casting. Once a casting design is fixed or finalized, alterations and modifications at a later stage to check formation of defects are difficult and costly. A good casting design implies a structure[107] which gives best service performance with least weight while still retaining a capability for being cast at good production rate. The purpose of a good casting design is to achieve functional performance of a structure at minimum cost in materials and manufacture. Simply, good service performance with cast ability should be combined in the design.

A good casting design is a contribution of not a one person but of a group of persons such as design engineer, foundryman, etc. A design engineer who is specialist of strength of the materials is more particular about load carrying ability of the part being designed. Hence, with his knowledge of the properties of materials and service stress analysis, he recommends a particular design of a part to be made of a suitable material. However, he is seldom wholly conversant with all features of the casting process which could be used for shaping the product design. On the other hand, a foundry engineer is mainly concerned with the castability of the design recommended and he decides a most economical method of the casting process to shape it. Hence, an ideal situation is to achieve close contact and cooperation between the design engineer and the foundryman so that latter's specific knowledge of founding could be used in the beginning stage of the design itself, before finalizing a design. Working together during the design stage, these two individuals can include in the design the most advantageous foundry features to make the part easier and cheaper to cast with reduced scrap loss and higher overall economy. Hence, of the various rules of the casting design, the very first rule is that the design engineer should consult the foundryman frequently as he designs a cast product and this collaboration between the two should occur in the beginning of the design only.

14.2 CASTING DESIGN ASPECTS AND PRE DESIGN CONSIDERATIONS

Broadly, there are two aspects of a casting design:[108-110]

1. **Engineering or Functional Aspect** i.e. to design a casting such that it successfully withstands the service requirement, for which it is intended.

2. **Foundry Aspect** i.e. without having any adverse effect on functioning of the part, to design or redesign the part for achieving casting soundness, dimensional accuracy and freedom from casting or cooling stresses at minimum cost.

Foundry design aspect and the measures adopted are thus concerned with the ease of moulding, with the problem of metal flow and feeding and with minimum stress generated during cooling of the casting. These factors collectively determine the soundness and dimensional stability of the casting.

Before committing to action for the design on the drawing board, the following can be taken into accounts for considerations:

1. Is it possible to delete certain members of the casting and weld them to the casting later to make foundry operations easier, cheaper and more dependable?
2. Should the casting be broken drown into component parts and separate component castings be welded together?
   The above two factors constitute what is known as **CAST-WELD DESIGN.**
3. Is the design such that the pattern can be adopted for economical moulding by standard methods?

4. Can risers, gates, and chills, etc. be positioned properly to ensure casting soundress?
5. Are the section size and configuration of the casting such as to cause undue stresses in the casting and consequent tearing or fracture of the casting?
6. Is it possible to establish and control directional solidification needed for casting soundness?
7. Can the model making be an aid in the desired casting design?

The last factor is an important consideration in case of complicated castings. In such cases, it is often desirable to make a model of the desired casting to determine accurately whether standard moulding methods can be adopted and whether it is possible to obtain sound metal in all critical areas.

Both the trouble and money could be saved, if an accurately scaled wood or plastic model can be made because even with the very competent foundry and/or design engineer, it is possible to miss many of important details as outlined above of the design when all that he sees is a blueprint of the design.

Many costly design changes and casting repairs can be avoided by making and studying a model of the job to be done. Areas of potential shrinkage defects, hot tearing can be predicated, gates and riser positions can be judiciously decided without trial and error and more serious changes in the casting design can be spotted before final working patterns are made.

For above modeling work, transparent plastics are excellent materials. Modeling clay can be also used to simulate padding and other features needed

14.3 SEQUENCE OF CASTING DESIGN

For very intricate castings and even for the simple castings, it is preferred to adopt the following design sequence:[111-112]

1. Establish the service conditions for casting from the layout and otherall specifications of the casting design.
2. Determine the static and dynamic forces and other critical requirements.
3. Layout the structural skeletons.
4. Decide the suitable composition of the iron to be used.

5. Check the stresses in terms of the iron selected.
6. Determine the general appearance of the casting from the point of view of its utility and sales appeal.

The foundryman opinions then can be sought on the suitability of this design with respect to moulding, soundness and cost of production. The foundryman can evaluate the above design and its successful production in the following sequence:

(*a*) Study the functions and arrangements required from the drawings prepared.
(*b*) Prepare isometric or perspective sketches or scaled model of the design, if required.
(*c*) Decide the parling line and the method of the pattern manufacture. Decide if any cores needed can be avoided or the moulding method can be simplified at this stage itself.
(*d*) Select the foundry method to be adopted with the gating and risering to be used. Decide the necessity of any pads, ribs, cored holes, etc. to be used or removed in consultation with the designer.
(*e*) Estimate the overall cost of production considering the rejections expected and the inspection methods to be adopted.

The details of the moulding method to be adopted and coring to be used should be carefully studied at this stage to achieve best results at economic cost. The application of the quality control method to be adopted during production should be considered rather than using it as a tool for distinguishing between good and bad castings during inspection as it can be an important factor in reducing the costs. The efforts should be of preventive nature and not for after cure.

14.4 CONSIDERATIONS FOR PRODUCTION ECONOMY

Changes in casting designs may be required not only by considerations of the quality of the product alone but by considerations of production economy as well. Variations in pattern making, moulding, core making, etc. must be thoroughly investigated to ensure most economical plan for producing castings of specified quality. The aim should be to bring modifications in the design of casting so that cost of all necessary operations in the production of casting is reduced to minimum without sacrifice of quality or changing the purpose of the original design.

Some of the important economic design considerations are:

14.4.1 Design for Pattern Making

1. Decisions should be made at the pattern making stage to determine best positions of the parting line and general approach to moulding and core making.
2. Pattern design should incorporate all necessary pattern allowances including moulding taper or draft for easy withdrawal of the pattern, shrinkage allowances, machine finish allowances, etc. Typical pattern shrinkage allowances are given in Table 14.1 for different iron castings depending upon pattern size and section thickness.[113]
3. Usually more pattern draft is necessary for hand moulding than machine moulding. Interior draft should be greater than exterior draft for easy removal of pattern as given below:

   Exterior draft–10 to 25 mm/meter
   Interior draft–40 to 65 mm/meter

4. Pattern should be sufficiently strong to resist warpage during moulding or pattern draw and also when stored.
5. For better casting surface finish, the pattern surface smoothness is an important factor. However, it maily depends on the sand surface or the casting process used as given in Table 14.2

14.4.2. Design for Moulding

1. Inorder to minimize moulding cost, aim should be to achieve a small mould volume and to employ minimum number of joints, cores and loose pieces.
2. Parting lines should be as few as possible and should preferably be completely flat as they are convenient and least liable to drops.
3. Moulds are most commonly cast with parting in horizontal plane since a vertically jointed mould requires special moulding boxes with special provision for access to runners and risers, etc.

TABLE 14.1: TYPICAL PATTERN SHRINKAGE ALLOWANCES.[113]

Type of metal	*Type of Construction*	*Pattern Size (inches)*	*Section Thickness (inches)*	*Contraction (inches/ft)*
Gray cast Iron	Open	Up to 24 (600mm)		1/8 (3.2mm/30cm)
	Open	25 to 48 (625-1200mm)		1/10 (2.5 mm/30cm)
	Open	Over 48 (1200 mm)		1/12 (2.0mm/30cm)
	Cored	Up to 24 (600mm)		1/8 (3.2mm/30cm)
	Cored	25 to 36 (625-900mm)		1/10 (2.5mm/30cm)
	Cored	Over 36 (900mm)		1/12 (2.0mm/30cm)
Malleable Iron			1/16 (1.56mm)	11/64 (42mm/30cm)
			1/8 (3.2mm)	5/32 (4mm/30cm)
			1/4 (6.2mm)	9/69 (3.5mm/30cm)
			1/2 (12.5mm)	7/64 (2.7mm/30cm)
			3/4 (18.2mm)	5/64 (2mm/30cm)
			1 (25mm)	1/32 (8mm/30cm.)
S.G. Iron				
Pearlitic		Up to 24 (600mm)		1/10 to 1/8 (2.5 to 3.2mm/30cm)
Ferritic		Up to 12 (300mm)		Nil

TABLE 14.2: SURFACE SMOOTHNESS OF CASTING.[113]

Casting Process	*Casting Finish, micro inches*
Green and casting	250-1000
Die casting	40-100
Precision casting	30-100
Plaster Casting	30

4. Any casting shape which makes pattern removal more difficult or moulding more complex should be avoided, if possible
5. Under cuts, reentrant angles, protruding bosses, flanges, etc. which are above or below the parting line require use of cores or loose pieces and should be avoided, if possible. Fig. 14.1. shows some of the improvements in the design which can make easier moulding.
6. Deep pockets are difficult to draw in green sand and they should be moulded in the drag so that the moulding sand does not hang down.
7. It is also desirable to have all or a greater portion of the mould cavity in the drag since it is easier to draw the pattern from the drag than to lift the cope off the pattern

14.4.3 Design for Coring

(*a*) Costs of mould construction with the use of cores are much greater than with mould alone. Hence, the possibility of elimination or reduction in coring in the mould should be explored.

(*b*) The cleaning problems are reduced and the overall economy as well as accuracy of the mould may be improved by decreasing the number of cores required.

(*c*) If used, the cores must be well supported with adequate size of core prints and chaplets to prevent shifting or raising and consequent casting inaccuracy.

(*d*) In general, a casting will be no better than its design allows the foundry to make it. Therefore, the simplification of the casting design should be explored to facilitate easier moulding and coring operations which in turn improve the production economy.

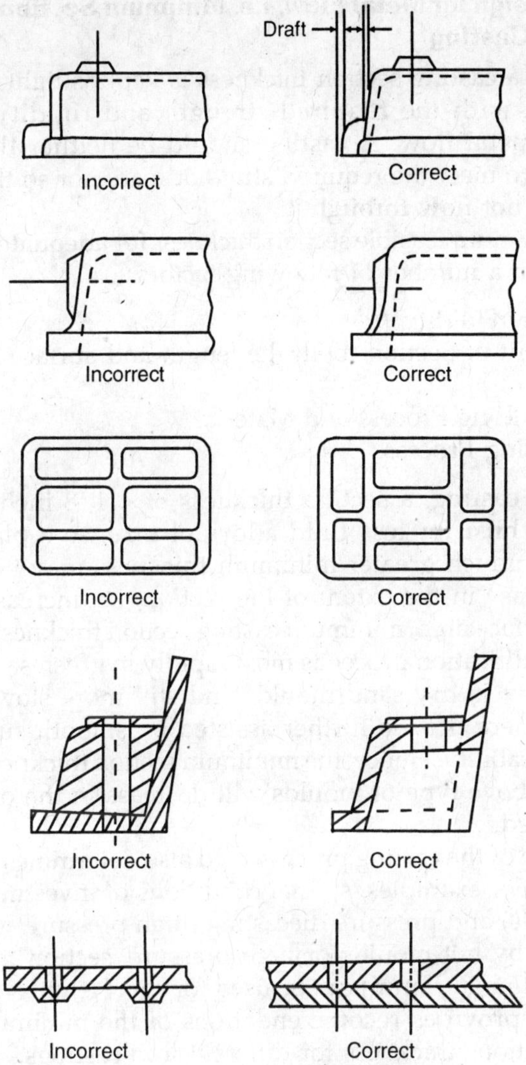

Fig. 14.1: Improvements in casting design[113].

14.5 CASTING DESIGN FOR ACHIEVING SOUNDNESS

The foundry aspect of the casting design in addition to above considerations, is also concerned with the problems of metal flow, feeding and subsequent cooling of the casting which collectively determine the soundness and dimension stability of the casting.

14.5.1 Design for Metal Flow, i.e. Minimum Section Thickness of Casting

Normally, a casting section thickness is kept as light as possible consistent with the required strength and rigidity and with required metal flow. A casting should be neither thicker than necessary to meet the required stress or load, nor so thin that the metal will not flow through it.

The minimum feasible section thickness for adequate metal flow depends on a number of following factors:

1. Alloy Fluidity.
2. Extent of Section (both the length and surface area of the section)
3. Moulding Process and Material
4. Casting Process.

In sand casting, a section thickness of < 1/8 inch (3 mm) is unusual whilst for less fluid alloys or extensive plate casting sections, a much greater minimum thickness may be required. With increase in the extent of the section, i.e. increasing length and/or surface area, minimum casting section thickness increases.

The solidification proceeds most rapidly in green sand moulds, more slowly in dry sand moulds and still more slowly in shell moulds where flow is further assisted by smooth surfaces and high permeability. Hence, the minimum section thickness required for these above type of moulds will decrease in the order of the mould listed.

The type of the casting process used also determines the section thickness. For examples, special conditions of investment casting (hot moulds) and pressure diecasting (high pressure) where flow is assisted by hot moulds or high pressure, section thickness as small as 0.15 in (0.4 mm) can be used for short lengths of castings. Table 14.3 provides recommendations of the minimum casting wall or sections thickness for different iron castings.

The above values are only a guide as many other factors are also involved Gray iron castings may chill to white iron if extended sections of 1/8 inch are used. Similarly, sections of under 1/2 inch may be too hard for machining with low carbon equivalent metal. Further, thin sections can be cast without misrun only if the distance from a larger section or runner is within limits. In general, sand castings of gray iron should not have < 1/8 in thick section for small castings, nor< 3/16 to 1/4 in for large castings.

TABLE 14.3: MINIMUM CASTING SECTION THICKNESS FOR IRON CASTINGS[110]

Type of casting	*Type of Alloy*	*Section thickness*
Sand casting	Gray cast iron	1/8-1/4 in (3.2-6.2mm)
	Malleable cast iron	1/8 in (3.2mm)
	White cast iron	1/8 in (3.2mm)
Gravity Die casting	Gray cast iron	3/16 in (4.8mm)
Investment casting	Gray cast iron	0.25-0.05 in (0.6-1.3mm)

14.5.2 Design for Soundness or Feeding (i.e. Avoiding or Minimizing Shrinkage Defects)

The lack of metal soundness in a casting is one principal reason for lower than optimum mechanical properties. Although the foundryman by the of special devices like gating, risering, chills, padding, etc. can generally produce sound castings even in very difficult cases of poorly designed castings, the job of producing required soundness and uniform good mechanical properties can be made easier and less costly, if certain following design principles are observed.

Generally, unsound castings having shrinkage cavities result due to presence of hot spots in their section thicknesses. These shrinkage defects are likely to occur in locations of extra mass known as "Hot Spots" which by means of their additional mass are the last portions in the section to solidify. They are those portions of the casting which cool more slowly than the rest.

A simple method to find out the locations of such extra masses (hot spots) is the use of Heuver's Inscribed Circle Method. This is based on inscribing largest possible circles within the boundary of the casting sections and measuring the radii of such circles. The following may be some of the examples of the locations of hot spots in casting sections:

1. Intersections or junctions of uniformly thick sections.
2. Intersections or junctions of sections of sharply differing cross sections.
3. Isolated concentrations of mass such as Bosses. Hubs, Pads, lugs, etc.
4. Heavy sections connected to risers by way of thinner or long sections.
5. Deeply recessed pockets.

14.5.2.1 Design of Junctions of the Uniform Sections

Usually, it is neither convenient nor economical to place a riser at hot spots of the junctions formed by the casting sections and it is necessary to rely upon feeding through one or more of the sections from a riser placed at some distance away. Since the sections are smaller, they will naturally freeze before the junction area, thus cutting of the supply of the feeding metal and the shrinkage will develop at the junction. Hence, there is need for modification of design of such junctions.

There are five basic types of junctions of uniform sections, typically represented by the letters, L, T, V, X, and Y as shown in Fig. 14.2. All other configurations at the corners could be considered modifications of one or more of these five letters. Hence, there are three types of junctions:

1. Junctions of two sections (L & V)
2. Junctions of three sections (T & Y) and
3. Junctions of 4 sections (X)

In general, the heat from metal is transferred in the mould in a direction perpendicular to the interface or radially, if the interface is curved. At the outer surface of the junctions, there is more mould meterial available to absorb the heat from the molten than is available adjacent to the straight protions of the casting that are well away from the corner. Consequently, the metal at this part of the junction will cool at some what faster rate than with the metal in the remote straight sections of the casting. Similarly, the metal at the inside corner of the junction will cool at much slower rate than the metal at the outside corner or in the straight areas because there is much less mould material available to absorb the heat of the molten metal. As a result, the metal in the junction near the inside corner surface will be the last to solidify and will be cut off from the feed metal, if the hot metal source is through the straight section of the casting and hence the shrinkage cavity will develop as shown in Fig. 14.2.

The principle of the modification of the design of such junctions is based on the fact that adequate fillet or radius is provided at such corners maintaining uniform wall thickness at the junction so that shrinkage cavity developed will become smaller because of increased cooling surface of the inner corner. Use of cored hole in these junctions will also reduce the mass of the metal to cool in these areas and hence will reduce the size of the defect formed or may eliminate its formation. But it is a doubtful solution. A solid casting without formation of any such defect is obtained by designing the section at the junction slightly smaller than of the straight arms and using an adequate inside radius. The above principles have been used in the design of the junctions formed as shown in Fig. 14.2. In the case of X-type junctions, off-setting one arm is the worse design as too rapid heat transfer between the junctions will occur which will increase the size of the defect formed. Therefore, the two arms should be offset considerably which can permit the use of chills and/or decrease in the size of the junction effectively to produce the solid casting. There has to be an optimum distance between the junctions formed by offsetting the arms as shown in the example of design of X-junction.

It should be emphasized that even if the designer is unable to design a joint which will not be free of shrinkage cavity, but he can design it such that it will have smallest possible defect formed and with such a design, the foundryman can easily apply his various methods of chilling, padding, directional solidification to produce a solid section. Thus, in general, out of all above 5 types of junctions of uniform sections, one should follow:

1. To attempt to limit such junctions formation;
2. To select the least difficult one and
3. To attempt to put minimum number of sections together.

14.5.2.2 *Design of Junctions of Unequal Sections and Sharply Differing Cross Sections*

Joints of dissimilar sections also produce shrinkage defects and contraction stresses like junctions of uniform sections but the contractions stresses formed at the junctions of unequal sections are of greater magnitude than in the cases of similar sections which cool relatively evenly. The stresses may be so severe that they can cause ruptures at these junctions.

The usual remedy for the feeding problem is taken care by placing riser at one end of the thick section and section proportioning for regulating solidification of the junction from where the thinner section can draw its feed metal. It is also advisable to incorporate a gradual increase in the thickness of the thinner section so that it is almost equal in thickness with the

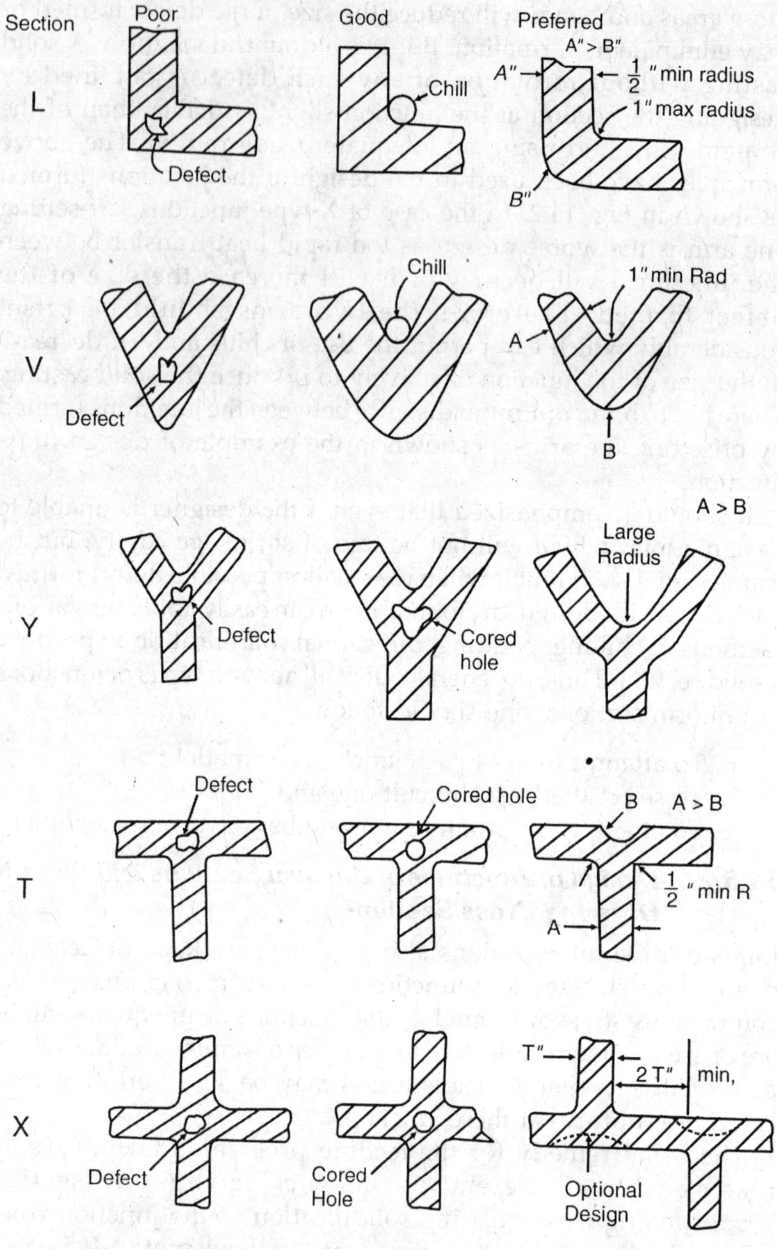

Fig. 14.2: Design of junctions of uniform section[113].

heavier section at the point of junction. Other general rules minimize stress concentration at the junctions are:

1. Adequate fillet radii should be provided in corners to reduce local stress generation but it should not be too large to create formation of the shrinkage defects.
2. Abrupt changes in section should be avoided and the principle of section blending (Fig. 14.3) should be adopted
3. Hot tear formation can be prevented and stiffening against distortion can be assisted by use of additional ribs, webs or tiebars (reinforcing agents). However, the thicknesses of such reinforcements should not be more than 2/3 of the parent section and the intersection effect produced by adding such ribs, webs can be reduced by coring out at the root of the reinforcing member.

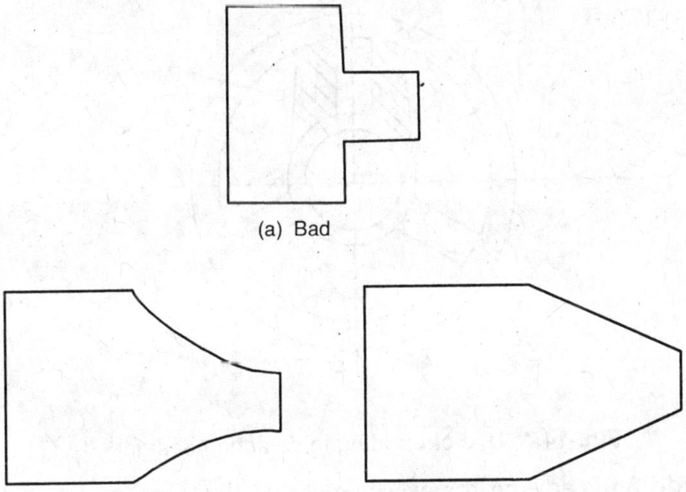

(a) Bad

(b) Fair

(c) Good

Fig. 14.3: Abrupt changes in casting section

14.5.2.3 Design for Achieving Directional Solidification

The use of directional solidification of the casting is normally applicable to eliminate formation of the centre-line shrinkage which usually occurs in case of steel castings. This defect in iron castings is only slightly trouble some and occurs particularly in low carbon equivalent gray irons or in malleable irons. The elimination of the centre-line shrinkage requires that there be a definite temperature difference in the casting between those portions furthest and those nearest the risers so that the directional solidification occurs towards the source of feedmetal (i.e. riser). This can be obtained either by tapering the casting or by use of padding such that a positive temperature gradient is set up towards the riser.

In case of tapering, the casting section is tapered to become larger towards the riser so that the temperature gradient will exist and the heavier portion of the casting will feed the thinner portion and the former can be in turn fed by the riser.

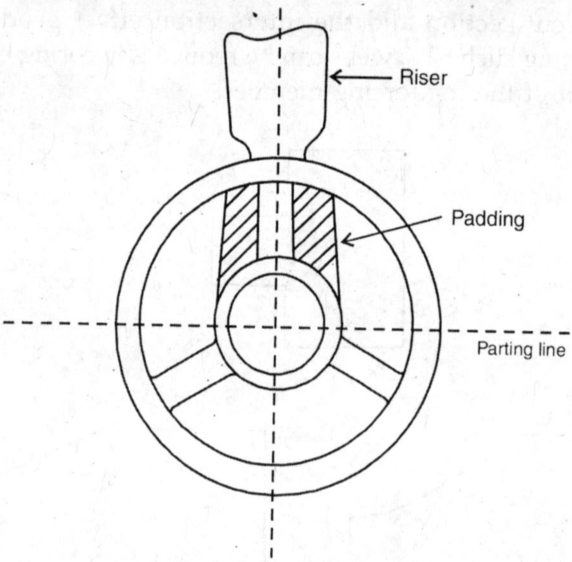

Fig. 14.4: Use of padding in a casting design[113].

Padding is adding the excess metal to the casting section (Fig. 14.4) such that its thickness increases towards the riser and thus setting up the temperature gradient needed for the directional solidification. This device should be used only when a taperred section is not desirable or permissible. This is because the pad metal is to be removed from the casting by chipping or by other method which is often an expersive method.

15

Gating and Risering of Iron Castings

15.1 INTRODUCTION

In making a casting, its design (shape and size) is determined based on the principles of so-called 'casting design' which takes into account its functional or service requirements and the foundry requirements, i.e. the castability. However, for making a quality casting i.e. a sound and defect free casting, there are certain other components or parts which are also required to be moulded and attached to the main casting cavity (mould) before pouring the casting although after solidification they are removed from the casting to constitute the so-called 'foundry return' of the casting which is used for remelting. These additional parts perform certain important functions and constitute Gating and Risering System of the casting. They are required even if only one casting is to be made and the volume of the metal lost in making these components decrease the casting yield. The design of these parts is therefore of paramount importance and is very carefully prepared to ensure production of a sound casting at an economical cost. This chapter will be devoted to design of such systems starting first with the design of the gating system followed by riser design or risering of the casting.

15.2 GATING DESIGN OF A CASTING

Gating or gating system of a casting refers to the system of the channels or passage ways which introduce liquid metal into the mould. Gates are the means to carry liquid metal from pouring ladle to the mould cavity. The design of these channels is based on certain fundamental principles of metal flow and is so important that there can be some times 30 to 40% of the casting rejection due to faulty gating design alone. A number of casting defects such as misruns, cuts, washes, slag and dross inclusions, scabs, trapped gases leading to gas holes, etc. may form due to a defective gating design. For example, an undersize gate will admit liquid metal into the mould at a jet velocity causing mould and core erosion and thereby sand inclusions in the casting besides other damages. On the other hand, an oversize gate will easily carry aspirated and trapped gases and slag along with the metal into the mould cavity. Therefore, an optimum size and design of gating is a must for quality casting production.

The gating design for a particular casting depends upon the following factors:

1. Type of metal or alloy being cast
2. Type of the casting process used
3. The design of the casting (shape and size of the casting)
4. Production requirements

15.2.1 Components of Gating System

The gating system used for a casting may consist of one or more of the following components as shown in Fig. 15.1.

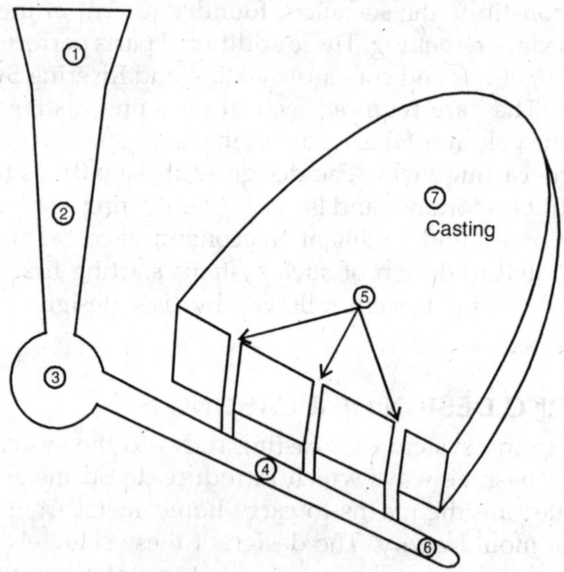

Fig. 15.1: Parts of a gating system: (1) pouring cup or pouring basin, (2) sprue or down sprue, (3) sprue base, button or well, (4) runner or cross gate, (5) gates or ingates, (6) runner extension

1. Pouring Cup or Pouring Basin
2. Sprue
3. Sprue Base, Button or Well
4. Runner or Cross Gate
5. Gates or Ingates
6. Runner Extension

In short, the functions of these different parts of a gating system are as follows.

1. **Pouring Cup or Basin:** To receive liquid metal and act as a reservoir. It also keeps liquid metal clean by preventing the entry of dross and slag in the remaining parts of the gating system and mould cavity.

2. **Sprue:** It takes metal vertically downward to rest components of gating system and thus provides the driving force (hydraulic head) along with the pouring cup or basin for controlling the flow rate of the metal into different components.

3. **Sprue Base:** It is an enlargement or rounded section provided at the bottom of the sprue to avoid turbulence generated due to high velocity of metal falling and also due to sudden change in the direction of the flow of metal from vertical to horizontal.

4. **Runner:** It is the second channel usually horizontal which distributes the metal around the mould cavity.

5. **Gates:** They are the third channel components which connect immediately into the mould cavity and by virtue of their design finally control the mould filling rate.

6. **Runner Extension:** This refer to the extended part of the runner beyond the last gate which is intensely moulded to trap the first flush of the cold and oxidized metal travelled through the other part of the gating system and thereby preventing its entry into the proper casting cavity through the gates.

15.2.2 Functions of an Ideal Gating System

It has been generally accepted[114-117] that an ideal gating system should perform the following functions:

1. To fill the mould cavity at a rate fast enough to complete the mould filling before premature freezing of the casting takes place.
2. To avoid or reduce agitation and thereby prevent the production of dross and its passage into the casting. It should also be capable of preventing dross or slag present in the ladle from reaching the mould.
3. To avoid the aspiration or entrainment of the air or mould gases in the metal stream.
4. To prevent mould and core erosion.
5. To aid in obtaining suitable thermal gradients to attain directional solidification and minimize distortion in the casting.
6. To avoid the necessity for high pouring temperature.
7. To afford maximum casting yield.
8. To provide case of moulding, pouring, etc. utilizing available facilities (i.e. it should be of simple design so as to facilitate moulding using mechanical methods and pouring using available ladle and crane equipments).

Many of above functions are conflicting with each other and a compromise is made between quality and economic requirements. The end result of any gating design should be to produce a saleable casting, i.e. a quality product at an economic price. In brief, the aim of a gating system is to permit entry of the liquid metal into mould cavity at a proper rate, without excessive temperature loss, free from objectionable turbulence, entrapped gases, slag and dross as well as mould and core material. Thus, metallurgically, a gating system should be such that it neither damages the metal, nor the mould.

15.2.3 Nature and Rates of Metal Flow

It has been established[114,115] that the flow of the molten metal follows the same principles as of hydraulic or water flow. However, the requirements of a gating system are opposite of those of a hydraulic system. In the latter case, every effort is made to reduce all frictional and kinematic losses to minimum so as to conserve power. In designing a gating system for a casting the reverse is the case, i.e. various kinds of losses are introduced so that the metal entering the mould has the lowest possible velocity and yet it should fill up the same at a rate fast enough before the loss of the temperature renders this impossible.

15.2.3.1 *Nature of Metal Flow*

Like any fluid, the liquid metal should flow either in a streamlined laminar fashion or in a turbulent manner as shown in Fig. 15.2.

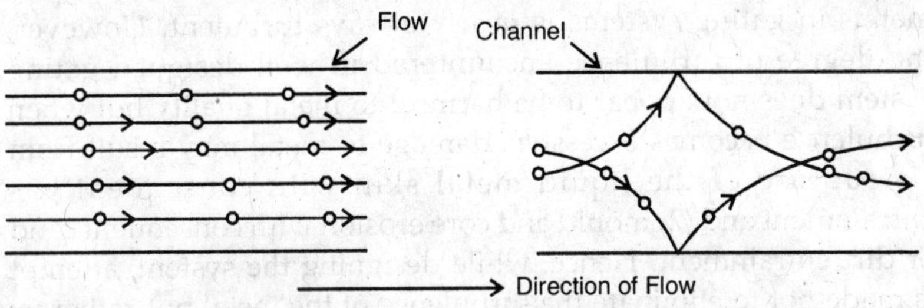

(*a*) Laminar or Streamlined Flow (*b*) Turbulent Flow

Fig. 15.2: Types of metal flow

In laminar flow, the particles of the fluid proceed smoothly parallel to the direction of flow. The velocity of the particles in a direction perpendicular to the direction of flow is therefore nil. Such flow occurs at low velocities. At high velocities, turbulent flow occurs. This is characterized by irregular movement of the particles of fluid across the stream in addition to their movement in the direction of flow.

Whether smooth or turbulent flow will occur, depends upon several factors such as velocity of the liquid, the cross section of the flow channel and the viscosity of the liquid. Their relationship is expressed as the Reynolds number (Rn) as given below:

$$Rn = \frac{v \times D}{\nu}$$

where, v = Mean velocity of flow

D = Diameter of the flow channel

ν = Kinematic viscosity of the liquid

Further, $\nu = \frac{\mu}{\rho}$

where, ρ = Density of the liquid

μ = Dynamatic viscosity of the liquid

Substituting the values of v in above equation

$$Rn = \frac{\rho.v.D}{\mu}$$

At low velocities when Rn < 2000, true streamlined flow occurs, whereas when Rn > 2000, flow is usually turbulent and this occurs at high velocities. The value of Rn varies in the range of 2000 to 20,000 for different types of metal flow in a gating systems[115,116,118] and hence, in classical hydrodynamic sense, the flow of liquid metals in gating systems is nearly always turbulent. However, the degree of turbulence encountered in well designed gating system does not appear to be harmful to metal quality but when turbulence becomes excessive, damage to metal may result from (1) rupture of the liquid metal skin with consequent gas entrainment and (2) mould and core erosion with consequent sand or dirt entrainment. Hence, while designing the system, attempt is made not to eliminate the turbulence of the metal but rather its reduction to a point when it is not harmful.

15.2.3.2 Rates of Metal Flow

The rates of metal flow through various gating parts is based on certain basic laws of the fluid flow. These are:

1. **Law of Continuity:** Which states that the flow rate must be the same at a given time in all portions of a fluid system. In the equation form, it may be expressed as

   $$Q = A_1 \cdot v_1 = A_2 \cdot v_2$$

   where Q = Flow rate
   and A_1 and A_2 are cross sectional areas of flow channel at two different portions 1 and 2.

   and v_1 and v_2 are the corresponding metal velocities of these two portions.

   This means that if the flow channel narrows down to half its original cross section, the metal velocity would be double and vice versa. However, the above law applies for completely filled channels.

   The second equation of the importance for metal flow is known as the Bernoulli's Theorem which is based on the first law of thermodynamics, i.e.

2. **Law of Conservation of Energy:** It states that the energy of a liquid of unit weight at a given point of the fluid system can be separated into three parts:

(*i*) Energy of velocity or kinetic energy = $\frac{v^2}{2g}$

(*ii*) Energy of Pressure or Pressure Energy = P/ρ and

(*iii*) Energy of Position or Potential Energy = h

where v is the velocity of the liquid, P is the static pressure in the liquid, ρ is the density of the liquid and h is the height of the liquid from a reference point.

In the ideal case (i.e. with no energy losses of any kind), when the liquid moves from point 1 to point 2, it neither gains, nor loses the energy. Thus, setting the energies equal for the two positions, yields the equation as given below:

$$\frac{v_1^2}{2g}+\frac{P_1}{\rho}+h_1=\frac{v_2^2}{2g}+\frac{P_2}{\rho}+h_2=constant$$

where v_1 and v_2, P_1 and P_2 and h_1 and h_2 are the corresponding values of velocity, static pressure and height of the liquid at two positions. These energies are convertible into each other.

The above equation (Bernoulli's Theorem) can be employed to calculate metal velocities only in ideal fluid system i.e. in systems in which the fluid suffers no energy losses. However, in real gating systems used, besides losses due to friction, energy losses also occur at all entrances and exits, bends, enlargement and contractions of the flow channel. The exit velocity and the flow rate obtained by the above equation would therefore, be somewhat higher than those found in actual practice. The Bernoulli's equation must be therefore modified to take the various losses into account as:

$$\frac{v^2}{2g}+\frac{P}{\rho}+h+h_2=Constant$$

where h_2 represents the total head loss and depending upon configuration of the gating system may be expressed as:

$$h_2=k_e\cdot\frac{v_e^2}{2g}+f\cdot\frac{\ell}{D}\frac{v^2}{2g}+k_b\cdot\frac{v_b^2}{2g}$$

$$+k_{ex}\cdot\frac{v_{ex}^2}{2g}+k_{en}\cdot\frac{v_{en}^2}{2g}+k_{con}\cdot\frac{v_{con}^2}{2g}+\ldots$$

where v_e, v_b, v_{ex} ... etc. are respective average velocities at point of losses.

k_e = entrance loss coefficient
f = friction loss coefficient
l = length of flow channel
D = Diameter of circular flow channel

$= \frac{4 \times Cross-sectinal\ area}{Perimeter}$ for other configuration

v = Average velocity in circular flow channel
k_b = bend loss coefficient
k_{ex} = exit or discharge loss coefficient
k_{en} = enlargement loss coefficient
k_{con} = contraction loss coefficient

If the gating system is completely filled during the metal flow, the velocities and the rates of the metal flow and hence, the pouring or mould filling time of the casting can be computed from the knowledge of the geometry of the gating system and the various loss coefficients.

For example, if v is the velocity of the metal flow at the gate calculated from the knowledge of the configuration and various loss coefficients of a gating design used and A is the total cross sectional area of the gate or gates, then the mould filling time, t can be obtained as:

$$t = \frac{V}{Q} = \frac{Volume\ of\ the\ casting\ poured}{Flow\ rate}$$

$$= \frac{W}{\rho \cdot A \cdot v}$$

where $Q = A \cdot v$
W = Weight of the casting poured (as it is easy to determine)
ρ = Density of the casting

For production of a quality casting, it is necessary that mould filling time is consistent and it does not vary from mould to mould of the same size. There is also danger of the loss of fluidity of the metal and hence, chances of premature freezing of the casting, if a consistent, predetermined mould filling time is not maintained.

15.2.4 Types of Gates and Gating Systems

Design of a gate (its size, shape and location with respect to main casting cavity) and its dimensional relationship with other parts of the gating system i.e. sprue and runner are very important considerations for successful production of casting.

15.2.4.1 Types of Gates

On the basis of the position with respect to the casting cavity, gates are of three types:

1. Top Gates
2. Bottom Gates
3. Parting Line Gates

15.2.4.1.1 Top Gates: In such cases of gates, metal enters through top of the casting [Fig. 15.3 (*a*)]. Such gates are usually limited to small sizes of the casting of simple design or large castings which are made in erosion resistant moulds. The latter is because of the fact that erosion of mould occurs as result of the turbulence of the metal entering the mould which also leads to gas entrainment. The mould erosion is a very severe problem in pouring of the cast irons and steels. Therefore, such gates are used in iron foundries for broad shapes or shapes of low depths of the castings.

Against the above limitations, there are also advantages of top gating. They are:

1. Such gates are simple to mould
2. Gates themselves may be made to serve as risers and hence, the casting yield increases.
3. Favourable temperature gradients are set up i.e. temperature increases from bottom of the casting towards the source of the hot metal i.e. riser. This situation promotes directional solidification.

15.2.4.1.2 Bottom Gates: They are most commonly used and the metal enters at the bottom of the casing [Fig. 15.3 (*b*)]. Therefore, very calm and quite entry of the metal takes place in the mould without much turbulence. However, such gates should be used along with side risers since the use of top risers creates unfavourable temperature gradient in the casting. Such gates are also difficult to mould and are made with the help of cores (additional items needed).

15.2.4.1.3 Parting Line Gates: The gates are moulded at the parting line of the mould cavity [Fig. 15.3 (*c*)]. These gates are the compromise between top and bottom gates and enjoy partial advantages of both these basic types and therefore, they are not the final solutions. However, they are easy to mould and can be moulded directly through the risers. Such gates are often chosen by the moulders since by moulding these gates at the parting line, various gating devices such as whirl gates, relief sprue, skim bob and choke etc. which help in filtering dross and slag can be easily adopted.

The above examples of the gates are those which are used as Single Gates for small size castings. However, for larger castings, several gates (known as Multiple Gates) are needed and used for pouring of the casting otherwise the mould material around the single gate, if used, will get excessively heated up and give rise to various sand expansion defects. Similarly, for large size castings, more than one runner may be also required while multiple gates are used.

The Multiple Gates are also of two types:

1. **Finger Gates:** They are horizontally disposed gating systems used for large size plate like castings.
2. **Step Gates:** They are vertically disposed gating systems used for the chunky castings. They are usually designed to take advantages of good features of the bottom gating and also correct their bad features.

15.2.4.2 Gating Ratio and Gating Systems

The dimensional characteristics of any gating system can be expressed in terms of what is known as 'Gating Ratio'. The latter is defined as the cross-sectional ratio of the sprue area (As) to the total runner area (Ar) to total gate area (Ag) i.e. As: Ar: Ag.

Depending upon the dimensional relationship between the different parts of a gating design, there are two types of the gating systems:

1. Pressurized Gating Systems
2. Un-pressurized Gating Systems.

15.2.4.2.1 Pressurized Gating Systems: In such gating systems, a back pressure is maintained on the gating components by a metal flow restriction provided at the gates. This usually requires that

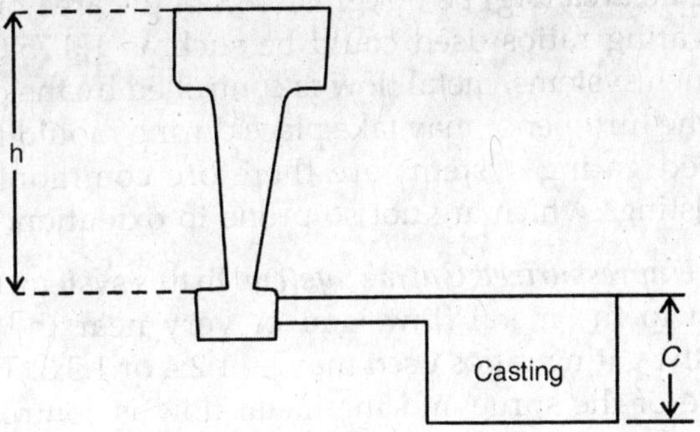

(*a*) Top Gates

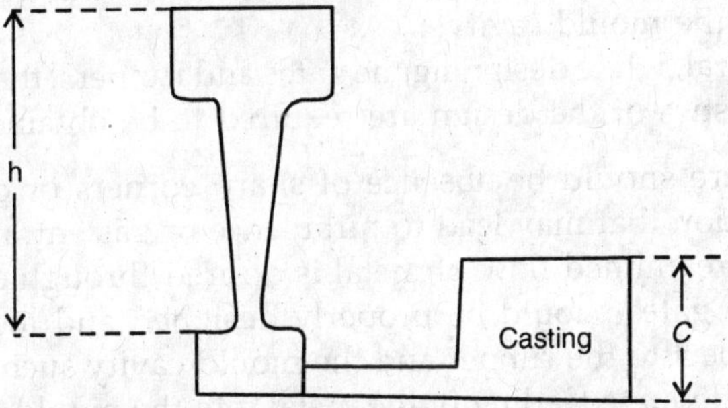

(*b*) Bottom Gate

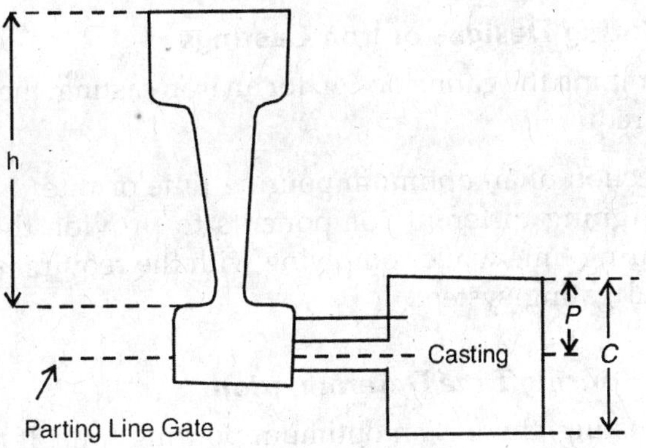

(*c*) Parting Line Gates

Fig. 15.3: Types of gates

the total gate area (Ag) be not greater than the area of sprue (As) e.g., the gating ratios used could be such as 1:0.75:0.5, 1:2:1 or 4:8:3. In such systems, metal flow is controlled by the choke at the gate and the turbulence may take place during mould filling. Such pressurized gating systems are therefore commonly used for ferrous castings which are not so prone to oxidation.

15.2.4.2.2 *Unpressurized Gating System:* In this system, the primary restriction to the metal flow is at or very near the sprue. For example, the gating ratios used may be 1:2:4 or 1:3:3. The choke is at the base of the sprue and the metal flow is controlled by the sprue area. Such gating systems are commonly recommended for light metal alloys such as aluminium or magnesium alloys which are prone to oxidation, since turbulence is reduced during metal flow into the mould cavity.

In general, while designing the gates and runners, the following characteristics of the design are required to be obtained:

1. There should be absence of sharp corners or changes of section that may lead to turbulence or gas entrapment, i.e. a streamlined flow of metal is desired through all parts.
2. The gates should be properly designed and located with respect to the runner and the mould cavity such that there is adequate feeding of the metal into the mould cavity and the flow rates are uniform through all gates.

15.2.5 Gating Designs of Iron Castings

For determining the gating design for an iron casting, the following steps are required:

1. Selection of an optimum pouring time or rate.
2. Designing different components to provide the selected pouring time while complying with the requirements of an ideal gating system.

15.2.5.1 Pouring Time Determination

For each casting, there is an optimum pouring time. If pouring is slower than the required optimum pouring time, the metal will freeze faster than before filling out the mould and the casting may develop cold metal defects. On the other hand, very rapid filling may cause erosion of the mould and core and other defects.

Based on Dietert extensive work for green sand moulding, the optimum pouring time for gray iron castings of different compositions has been determined as function of its thickness, weight and fluidity and is given by the equation[119,120]:

$$\text{Pouring time, } t(\text{sec}) = K\left(0.95 + \frac{T}{0.853}\right)\sqrt{W}$$

for casting weights not exceeding 450 kg.

$$\text{and Pouring time, } t(\text{sec}) = K\left(0.95 + \frac{T}{0.853}\right)\sqrt[3]{W}$$

for casting weights more than 450 kg.

where K is the fluidity coefficient or factor.

W is the weight of the casting in lb

and T is the average thickness of the casting in inches.

The value of the fluidity coefficient is obtained from the relations developed[121] as curves for spiral fluidity as a function of iron composition and pouring temperature. For shell-moulded and vertical pouring of S.G. iron casting, the optimum pouring time has been determined as[122]:

$$\text{The Pouring time, } t \text{ (sec)} = K\sqrt{W}$$

where K = 1.8 for 3/8 to 1 inch sections

= 1.4 for thinner sections

= 2.0 for heavier sections

15.2.5.2 Design of Gating Components

After the optimum pouring time has been established, the next step is to design the various parts of the gating system shown in Fig. 15.1. In general, attempt is made to design these parts with the aim of reducing turbulence, aspiration of gases, dross formation, mold and core erosion and preventing entry of the slag and other non-metallics from entering the mould cavity while incurring minimum wastage of metal and achieving low cost of production.

Pouring Cup or Basin: This is the first part which receives molten metal from the pouring ladle. The aim is to pour from a low height into the pouring cup or basin of adequate size which can maintain control of the metal flow and be deep enough to prevent vortex formation in the sprue. Most frequently, pouring cups are used as they are economical and simple to mould and various alternate designs of the same used in iron foundries are shown in Fig. 15.4 (*a*). However, pouring cups do not have control in checking the entry of slag and dross as well as on the flow rate of the metal and vortex formation leading to air or gas entrapment in the metal stream. Therefore, for quality castings, use of pouring basin as shown in Fig. 15.4 (*b*) is recommended in which the metal is poured into a chamber partitioned by the barcore which prevents the slag and dross from entering into the sprue and also delivers metal into the sprue under a constant pressure with the help of the dam moulded. The vortex formation is also reduced when the metal from the ladle do not directly fall over the sprue. The size of the basin is a function of the size of the casting poured and a rectangular shape is preferable to a circular one. A pouring basin stopper rod can be used while the basin is being filled and this ensures complete filling of the sprue and reduces the time taken to fill the remainder of the gating system. A radiused exit (with at least one inch radius) of the basin which should blend well into the sprue is recommended.

Sprue: The sprue height along with the height of the metal in the basin provides effective head (H) of the molten metal (the driving force) which governs the metal flow rate at the base of the sprue. This effective head of the molten metal varies depending upon the type of the gate employed. For example, as shown in Fig. 15.3, the effective head $H = h$ in top gating, $H = h - \frac{c}{2}$ in bottom gating and $H = 2hc - P^2/2c$ in parting line gating.

A large top end tapered sprue is recommended with the choke (restriction in the sprue cross section) at the base of the sprue which regulates to obtain the desired pouring rate. The taper must be sufficient to obtain a completely filled sprue to avoid mould gas aspiration. It is recommended[117] that the area of the top of the sprue should be twice the sprue choke area for short lengths of the sprue and three times the sprue choke area for tall sprues.

Sprue Base: This component minimizes the turbulence achieved by high velocity of the metal stream emerging form the sprue exit as well as from the change in direction of metal flow from vertical to horizontal. A cylindrical shape of the sprue base is recommended, approximately twice the runner width in diameter and extending slightly above and below the runner. The sprue should join the base with a small radius (say 1/8 inch).

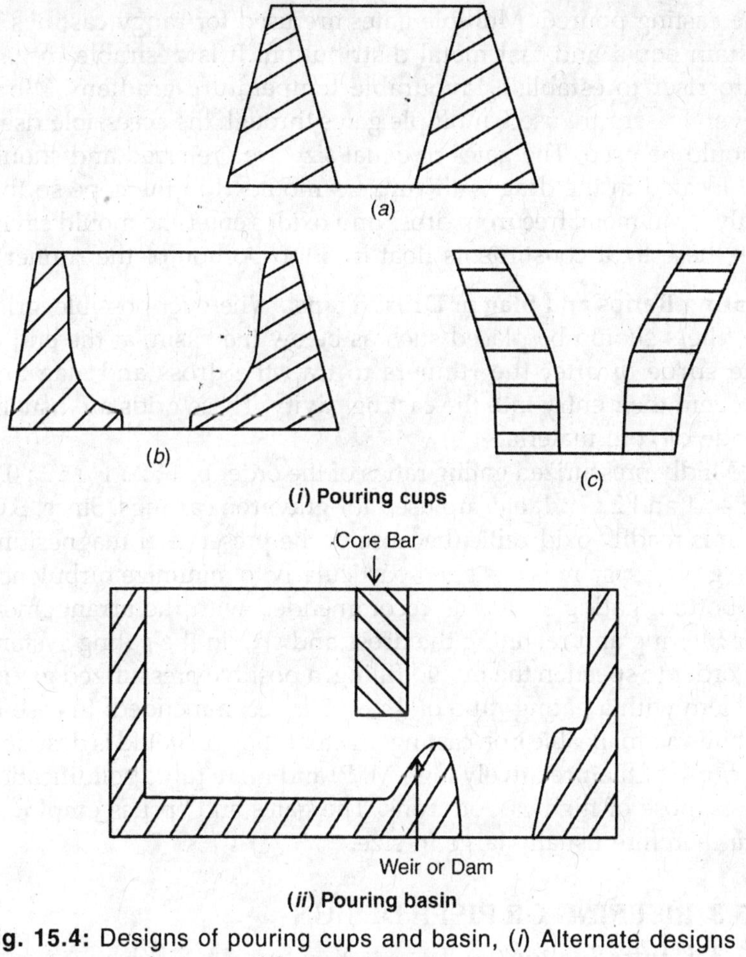

(*i*) **Pouring cups**

(*ii*) **Pouring basin**

Fig. 15.4: Designs of pouring cups and basin, (*i*) Alternate designs of pouring cups, (*ii*) pouring basin

Runners: This part distributes the molten metal around the mould cavity and also regulates the temperature gradient set-up in the casting. It is made approximately four times larger in cross-sectional area than the bottom of the sprue. On use of multiple gates, the cross sectional area of the runner is reduced past each ingate by an amount depending upon the gating ratio used to maintain uniform flow of the metal from each ingate. The runner is prepared by firmly rammed good quality moulding sand.

Ingates: The number of ingates used depends upon the size of the casting poured. Multiple gates are used for rangy castings to obtain equal and fast metal distribution. It is desirable to gate into riser to establish favourable temperature gradient. When several risers are used, multiple gates through the accessible risers should be used. The gates of equal size are preferred and should be located in the drag with runners moulded in the cope so that only clean metal free from dross and oxides enter the mould cavity (as these light constituents float into top portion of the runner).

Gating Ratios and Slag or Dross Traps: Wherever possible, grids or filters should be placed such as below the basin, at the end of the sprue or after the runners to trap the dross and slag and prevent their entry into the casting cavity. These grids are usually made of core materials.

Mildly pressurized gating ratios of the order of 1 : 2 : 1, 1 : 2 : 0.5, 1 : 4 : 1 and 2 : 7 : 1, etc. are used for gray iron castings. Since, S.G. iron is readily oxidizable (because of the presence of magnesium) the gating system is designed particularly to minimize turbulence. A bottom gating system is recommended with the arrangement for filtering and retaining the dross and slag in the gating system. In order to speeden the mould filling, a positive pressurized gating system with a gating ratio of 4 : 8 : 3 is recommended. In case of white and malleable iron castings, faster filling of mould is desirable because of their relatively high M. P. and more rapid solidification than those of high-carbon irons. The gates and sprues employed are therefore usually large in size.

15.3 RISERING OR RISER DESIGN

15.3.1 Introduction

Risering is a process designed to prevent the formation of shrinkage voids in a casting upon solidification. Castings of heavy sections or of high-shrinkage alloys commonly require a riser or reservoir where metal can stay as liquid while the casting is freezing. According to the definition given by the Gating and Risering Committees of the American Foundrymen's Society[123-125], a Riser (also variously called as Feeder, Header or Feedhead) is a reservoir connected to the casting for the purpose of feeding liquid metal to the casting during solidification, to offset the shrinkage which takes place while the casting is solidifying. Sometimes, simple risers are used whose function is to allow escape of the mould gases and provide extra metallostatic pressure forcing the liquid to reproduce the mould details completely. However, as most casting metals and alloys contract while freezing, the application of feeders is more general than that of simple risers.

Various investigations on solidification of metals have demonstrated[125-127] that the absolute density of a casting (having zero porosity) is unattainable and therefore, generally, castings are rejected on the basis of the presence of the macroshrinkage rather than on the basis of microshrinkage whose control is generally uneconomic. Hence, the aim of feeding a casting is a not to attain absolute casting density but to see that microshrinkage is uniformly distributed and not concentrated at heat centres. Thus, the feeding of castings has been defined as the process of compensating for volumetric contraction in such a way as to ensure that sound castings, free from or with a controlled amount of shrinkage cavities result.

15.3.2 Functions of Riser

The functions of a riser can be summarized[123] as follows:

1. To absorb volumetric contraction
2. To vent the mould cavity
3. To indicate when mould is full
4. To avoid straining of casting
5. To flow-off cold metal

1. The metals and alloys contract in three stages, out of which the volumetric contractions in the liquid stage and solidification stage are compensated by the feed metal of the riser. The amount of the liquid contraction varies with the melt super feet (~ 1.6% per 100° C melt super heat) but usually, this contraction is fed by the liquid metal flowing through the gating channels. The solidification contraction which occurs due to change in the state of the metal is quite considerable and varies with the nature and composition of the alloy.

For example, in case of cast irons, such volumetric contraction varies as given below.

White cast irons—4.0 to 5.50%

Gray irons—1.6% to negative value depending upon composition and expansion due to graphitization

In addition to above contractions (due to change in volume), a peculiar type of volumetric compensation has to be met by supply of feed metal from the riser in cases of cast irons such as gray and ductile irons which occurs due to a phenomenon known as Mould Dilation. The latter refers to expansion in volume of the mould which occurs in weak mould, particularly due to pressure developed within the casting as a result of graphitization occurring during solidification. As a result of it, the casting will bulge outward and large cavity will develop in the casting. If the mould is very weak, there could be mould dilation due to metallostatic pressure of the liquid metal itself. A volumetric mould cavity expansion of about 1.5% is generally obtained in a green sand mould. The effect of several variables including the compositions of the iron and sand mould on such Mould Wall Movement has seen studied in a great detail by Wallace and Evans[128]. The problem of mould dilation can be reduced by hard ramming, low moisture and sea coal additions in green sand moulds.

2. Riser also acts as vent (outlet) for escape of air and mould gases while metal is being poured. However, this function is of great importance in permanent moulds, dry sand moulds coated with impervious blacking and in green sand mould when permeability is low.
3. Riser also indicates when the mould is full. It is particularly important when the mould is poured by men other than who have prepared the mould (having no idea about the volume of mould being poured).
4. When the metal is moving at a fast rate during mould filling and suddenly it stops at the cope surface of the mould, the kinetic energy of the metal will be transformed into pressure energy which may throw out some metal if there are any openings available through vents or at the parting line, or otherwise the pressure energy developed will work over the solidifying casting and may strain it. On the other

hand, when the riser is attached to the casting, the liquid metal will continue to flow through it instead of suddenly stopping at the cope surface and thus the possibility of above event is avoided.

5. The riser also helps in flowing off the cold and oxidized metal through it which may otherwise remain within the mould cavity.

Some of the above functions are performed by a riser only when it is a open riser and not the blind one.

15.3.3 Requirements of Riser

In order to perform the main function of feeding the casting satisfactorily, there are certain technical and also economic requirements of a riser. They are:

1. **Feed Volume Criteria:** A riser must have sufficient volume of liquid metal to provide for compensation of different volumetric contractions occurring in the casting. Simply, this refers to the size requirement of a riser.
2. **Freezing Time Criteria:** The riser must freeze sufficiently slowly to ensure that liquid metal is available throughout the freezing of the casting. In other words, the solidification time of the riser should be greater than the casting.
3. **Placement Criteria:** The riser should be positioned at or adjacent to the thick or heavy section of the casting and should exploit factors favourable to feeding such as set up of proper temperature gradient, its own metallostatic pressure and in some cases, even atmospheric pressure.

The above three are considered as minimum requirements of a riser. In addition to these, it is desirable that a riser should be economic as well.

4. **Economic Criteria:** The riser should be so designed and placed that it will accomplish its mission with minimum wastage of metal and with maximum efficiency.

15.3.4 Riser Dimensioning And Placement

The riser design consists of determination of the following:

1. Shape of the Riser
2. Size of the Riser
3. Position of the Riser

15.3.4.1 Shape of a Riser

Determination of shape of a riser is based on the second requirement of the riser i.e. freezing time criteria–a riser should preferably solidify later than the casting. In 1940, *N.* Chvorinov developed an equation which related freezing time of a riser to that of the casting assuming that both riser and the casting are the two cast shapes. His equation of the freezing time of a cast shape is given by:

$$t\,(\textit{freezing time}) = K \cdot \left(\frac{V}{S}\right)^2$$

where

V = Volume of the cast shape
S = Surface area of the cast shape
K = Constant whose value depends on the pouring temperature, moulding material and composition of the alloy

He plotted a curve between freezing time (t) and V/S ratio of different shapes of a cast product of the same volume and found that a spherical shape gives longest freezing time, followed by the cylindrical shape, a cube and plate shape. Since riser must freeze sufficiently showly, any cast shape which gives maximum value of V/S will be the most desirable shape of a riser. Accordingly, a spherical shape is the most desirable shape of the riser. However, there are practical problems associated with the spherical shape of a riser. Spheres are usually difficult to mould and would present the feeding problem as well since the last metal to freeze would be near the center of the sphere, where it could not be used to feed a casting. Hence, the next best theoretical shape i.e. the cylinder is chosen as an ideal shape of the riser which does not suffer from limitations of a sphere. The cylindrical shape of a riser is thus most universally adopted and wherever is possible, to further maximize its V/S ratio, a hemi-spherical top of the cylindrical riser can be also used.

15.3.4.2 *Size of a Riser*

The size of a riser is determined on the basis of the first two requirements of the riser i.e. Feed Volume Criteria as well as Freezing Time Criteria, both of which must be satisfied.

A number of methods of riser size determination have been developed, of which a few are in applications for riser dimensioning. Attempt will be made here to briefly discuss the principles of some of these important methods.

1. **Chvorinov's Method:** This method was originally developed for determination of the size of a riser for steel casting and according to it, freezing time of a riser, $t_{riser(R)} \geq t_{casting(C)}$, freezing time of the casting.

   In other words, $\left(\frac{V_R}{S_R}\right)^2 \geq \left(\frac{V_C}{S_C}\right)^2$ i.e. the square of volume to surface area ratio of the riser must be greater or equal to that of the casting as value of the K is same for both. For any given casting whose V/S ratio is already known, various V_R/S_R of different sizes of a cylindrical riser are calculated and a riser whose $\left(\frac{V_R}{S_R}\right)^2$ value is little larger than of the casting–say 10 to 15% greater–is selected as the riser of the casting. However, this method is based only on the freezing time criteria as it does not take into account the feed volume requirement. Therefore, this method was found to be valid for only some simple and small size castings of steels and could not be universally used. However, this method is of historical importance as it provided a basis for a number of other important methods which are in use.

2. **Caine's Method:** In 1947, J.B. Caine was the first to adopt the first two basic requirements of a riser in his approach for developing a risering method for steel castings[129]. Elaborating Chvorinov's Rule, he developed an equation, $x = \frac{a}{y-b} + c$ which is also applicable to all metals for risering.

   where $y = \frac{V_S}{V_C} = \frac{\text{Volume of Casting}}{\text{Volume of Riser}}$

$$x = \text{Freezing Ratio} = \frac{\frac{S_C}{V_C}}{\frac{S_R}{V_R}} = \frac{\frac{\text{Surface Area of Casting}}{\text{Volume of Casting}}}{\frac{\text{Surface Area of Riser}}{\text{Volume of Riser}}}$$

b = Fractional Solidification Shrinkage

c = Relative Freezing Rate of Riser and Casting

a = Freezing Characteristic Constant

The plot between x an y gives a curve of a hyperbola and sound casting are obtained by choosing the values of x and y which give a point falling on the right side of the curve (Fig. 15.5).

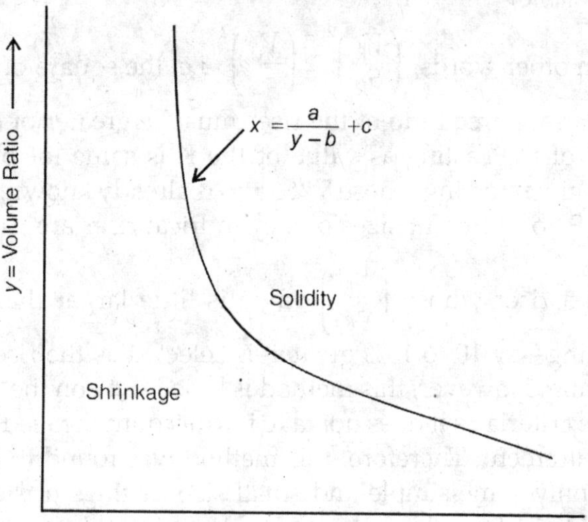

Fig. 15.5: J.B. Caine's risering curve

However, this method of risering involved a time consuming trial-and-error calculations to get the size of a desirable riser.

3. **Shape Factor or NRL Method:** A group of researchers working at Naval Research Laboratory[130], USA in 1955 modified the Caine's Method of riser dimensioning and substituted his Freezing Ratio by a Shape Factor, S to avoid the trial-and-error calculations, required. The Shape Factor is given by:

$$S = \frac{L+W}{T} = \frac{\text{Length} + \text{Width}}{\text{Thickness}} \text{ of the casting}$$

The values of L, W and T are computed by using the maximum dimensions of the parent section (i.e. when casting is made of heavy and light sections). The curve obtained by plotting y (Ratio of riser volume to casting volume) and shape factor values (x) is known as shape factor chart. They further found that the most economical height (h) to diameter (d) ratio of side risers is unity and that of the top risers is 0.5.

They also prepared a riser dimensioning chart by plotting the value of riser volume (obtained from the shape factor chart for a given size of the casting) and the riser height and diameter ratio falling between 1 and 0.5. This method was found to be simple for riser size determination (although less accurate than Caine's Method) and was used for steel castings as well as for alloys which solidify in skin formation manner including some S.G. cast irons.

4. **Wlodawer's Modulus Method:** This method was developed in 1963 by *R.* Wlodawer[131] who based his method on direct application of Chvorinov Rule and defined the term Modulus or Cooling Modulus of a Casting (Mc) as:

$$M_C = \frac{\text{Volume}}{\text{Surface Area}} \text{ of the casting with the modification}$$

that only cooling surfaces are to be considered and imaginary contact surfaces between riser and casting are omitted. To simplify modulus calculations, the principle of substitute bodies is employed and he has shown that for all complicated shapes of the casting, modulus can be calculated from using basic units like plates, bars and spheres.

According to him, the Modulus of the desired riser or feeder M_f can be obtained from the modulus of the casting by the relation as:

$$M_f = K \cdot M_C$$

where K = 1.2 (which takes care of both the feed volume and freezing time requirements)

The size of the riser then can be calculated from the value of Modulus of Riser assuming $H = D$ or $H = 1.5\ D$

where H = Height of Riser

and D = Diameter of Riser

This method has been found to be most comprehensive of all methods and is valid for all metals and alloys as well as different mould materials used.

15.3.4.3 *Location or Placement of a Riser and Feeding Distance*

Location of riser on a solidifying casting is a very important consideration from the point of view of feeding of the casting. The following should be considered:

1. The riser should be located with proper gating near or at the heaviest section of the casting which is last to solidify.
2. The location of a riser should be such that all the parts of the casting are within the Feeding Range or Distance of the Riser. There is a definite limit to the distance a riser can feed adequately even in a uniform section. This distance is called as Feeding Distance or Range of the Riser.
3. The location of the riser also should aim at setting favourable temperature gradient in the casting so that directional solidification takes place from the casting extremities towards the source of hot metal i.e. riser.

Large or complex castings require multiple (several) risers when sections of the castings lie out side the feeding distance of a riser. The number of risers thus selected should be such that the sections of the casting lie equally within the feeding range and maximum casting yield is obtained. The feeding distance of a riser is a function of the thickness of the casting section as well as other feeding aids which help in promoting set-up of the favourable temperature gradient in the casting.

15.3.5 Riser Designs of Iron castings

In gray iron castings, little risering is needed for the purpose of feeding shrinkage of such castings and sometimes, use of proper runner can solve the purpose of feeding the casting. However, risering becomes very critical for other requirements of riser such as mould wall movement which occurs both in gray irons and S.G. irons due to pressure developed by graphitization, particularly in case of weak sand moulds. This phenomena of mould dilation in soft and green sand moulds may produce an additional 15% feed metal requirement above that needed to satisfy the liquid and solidification[132] shrinkage. In such cases, stronger moulds are prepared and careful risering is needed.

The risering of gray irons depends upon many variables such as type of mould, composition of the metal and dimensions of the casting. A standard amount of mould wall expansion is considered even for a good quality green sand mould. The liquid contraction as well as solidification contraction are also considered while computing the size of the riser. The liquid contraction depends on the composition of the iron and melt superheat. The values for these two contractions have been measured.[132] For example, for gray irons it will be in the range of 0.68 to 1.8% per 100° C melt superheat. Similarly, the solidification shrinkage for such irons may very from 1.6% to negative value (2.5% expansion) depending on graphization.

Wallace and Evans[133] have developed a method of riser size calculation for different gray iron compositions in which both Caine's approach as well as NRL technique have been incorporated. They have used 1.5% as the amount of the mould wall expansion in green sand mould and zero% in dry sand mould and liquid and solidification contraction values as 2% and 0 to 1.4%, respectively for two types of irons (soft and high strength gray irons) chosen. Simplifying assumptions of Caine's and NRL methods and considering cylindrical riser with a height equal to diameter, they obtained an equation giving surface area of the casting (S_{AC}) as a function of volume of casting (V_C) and riser diameter (D) as:

$$S_{AC} = \frac{125}{\dfrac{D}{b \cdot V_C} - \dfrac{\pi}{4D^2}} = \frac{125}{\dfrac{D}{b \cdot V_C} - \dfrac{1.275}{D^2}}$$

where b = fractional solidification shrinkage.

Compositions of irons selected for this study were as follows:

Type of Irons	*%C*	*%Si*	*%P*	*%S*	*%Mn*
Soft gray Iron	3.5	2.2	0.05	0.10	0.60
High strength gray Iron	3.0	1.5	0.05	0.10	0.80

The values selected for mould wall movement and solidification contraction for the above irons were added to obtain the value of *b* in the above equation. The riser diameter *D* obtained from the above equation was adjusted to allow for 2% liquid contraction in the volume of the riser and the casting to get the final value of *D*. The results of these calculations have been plotted (as log-log plot) in Fig. 15.6 for high strength iron casting moulded in green sand and in Fig. 15.7 for high strength iron in dry sand mould and soft iron in green sand mould.

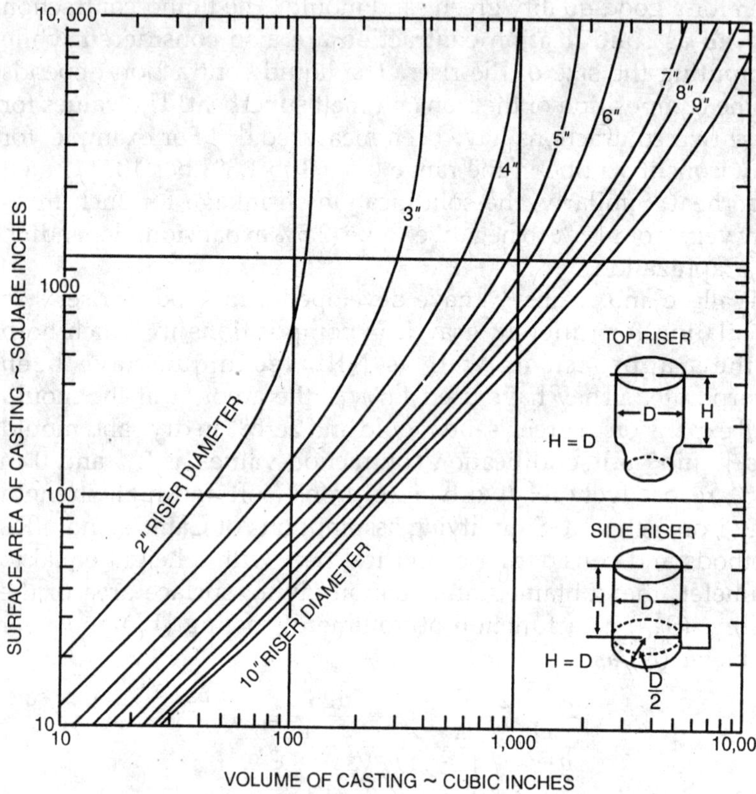

Fig. 15.6: Relation between surface area and volume of casting for high strength gray iron casting poured in green sand mould[133].

When multiple risers are required for a given casting, the size of riser is determined on the basis of the surface area and volume of that portion of the casting fed by this riser. In case of uniform sectioned castings, they are generally divided into equal portions for such computation of riser size with one riser for each section. However, for complicated (irregularly shaped) castings, the casting portions and the resulting risers may be of different sizes. In a recent past work, Turnbull, Merchant and Wallace have investigated[134] the values of feeding distance for gray iron castings which can be used in such cases and will help in deciding the number of risers required.

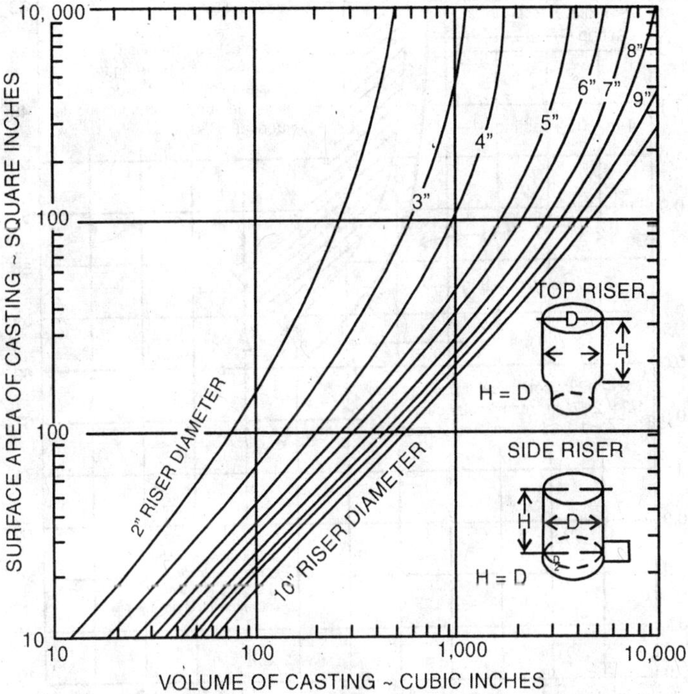

Fig. 15.7: Relation between surface area and volume of casting for high strength gray iron casting poured in dry sand mould and soft gray iron casting poured in green sand mould[133].

In case of S.G. iron castings, the change in graphite form from flakes type (in gray iron) to nodular is accompanied by major differences in solidification behavior. The precipitation of such graphite in nodular form causes in S.G. iron castings to expand to a greater degree and with more force than gray iron[135].

Consequently, they require more rigid moulds and greater care to feeding for getting a sound casting. The solidification shrinkage of such irons varies[132] from 2.7% (contraction) to 4.5% (expansion). In green sand moulds, S.G. iron castings are therefore likely to be much oversize compared with gray iron castings.

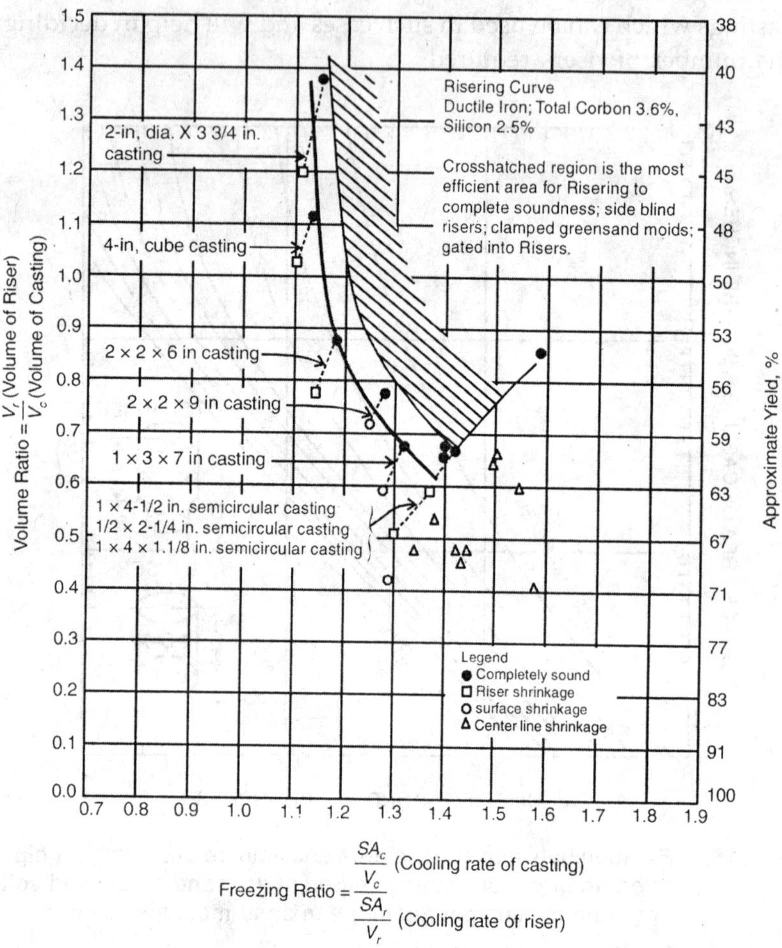

Fig. 15.8: Curve for calculating side blind risers for S.G. iron castings[136].

Flinn, Reese and Spindler have studied in greater detail[136] about the risering of the S.G. iron castings of different sizes. They have adopted Caine's Method directly for riser size calculation as:

$$\text{Freezing Ratio of } \frac{\text{Casting}}{\text{Riser}} = \frac{\dfrac{\text{Surface Area of Casting}}{\text{Volume of Casting}}}{\dfrac{\text{Surface Area of Riser}}{\text{Volume of Riser}}}$$

should be greater than one to get sound casting, since the cooling rate of the riser must be less than that of the casting in order to have liquid feed metal available while the casting is solidifying.

The ratio of volume of riser and volume of casting as well as the freezing ratio are then calculated and for a given casting-riser combination, these above two values establish a point in the curve (Fig. 15.8). For getting the sound casting, this point must lie to the right of the curve and preferably in the shaded area to obtain the maximum yield. Several trial-and-error calculations (usually two are sufficient) quickly establish the size of a cylindrical side riser having same height and diameter.

In order to know the number of risers required for a casting, these authors have also adopted the same approach as used for steel castings by Bishop and pelline[137].

Accordingly, for Plate casting, feeding distance = $4.5T$

and for Bar casting, feeding distance = $6\sqrt{T}$ are used.

where T is the thickness of the Plate/Bar Casting. The thickness of plate casting varied between 1/4 to 2 inches and that of the bar casting between 2 to 4 inches. These data may be projected for more complex shapes since all castings may be considered as combinations of such simple geometrical shapes. A cube may be also visualized as a very short bar.

The white iron has a relatively large solidification shrinkage which is relatively difficult to feed as the white iron solidifies in two stages. There is hardly any work which may provide information for the riser size calculation. However, Caine's method of riser dimensioning as well as feeding distance calculations as discussed above for S.G. iron castings can be used. The use of chills can further improve feeding distance by causing sharp temperature gradient in the casting.

16

Indian Practice of Cast Iron Technology

16.1 INTRODUCTION

Casting of metals and alloys is known through ages, from the days when prehistoric men acquired the knowledge of utilizing metals. However, the techniques of casting have undergone spectaculars changes over the centuries and the art of casting has given way to science quite long back. Castings are required by the entire manufacturing industries, be it the oil, textile, ship/building, automobile, aircraft, construction or agriculture industry. Casting has been, and will continue to be, the cheapest form of metal-forming technology. It is only by the foundry technology that the most intricate shapes can be formed, unlike the forging industry and the sheet-metal industry, which have limitations.

Metal casting in India is many centuries old and as evident from excavations at Mohenjodaro and Harappa, it dates back to 3300-2000 BC. Although founding started in this country with non-ferrous castings, the skill in ferrous castings is also quite old as evident from Ashok Pillars standing for hundreds of years. However, the metal casting in India as an industry (organized and producing castings on mass scale) started in the later part of the nineteenth century. Since then, the foundry has made rapid progress in all fields and today, India has expertise to make castings of all types and varied metallurgical compositions to meet the growing needs of different industries. The Indian foundry industry in the last decade has witnessed robust growth and India now ranks 6th as the largest casting producer in the world in tonnage and the second largest in total number of foundries[138, 139]. An attempt will be made in this chapter to present an outline of the present status of the Indian foundry industry dealing with the impact of the economic policy reform of the government on expansion and modernization of the existing units, in general, and in particular, details of the casting technologies of the various cast iron foundries, their some of the problems and possible remedies and the future challenges to be faced and lines of actions to be taken.

16.2 PRESENT SCENARIO AND RECENT TRENDS OF INDIAN FOUNDRY INDUSTRIES

For historic reasons, Indian Foundry industry is a unique blend of old and new. The foundry as a craft and foundry as a technology have curiously co-existed in the country and have progressed to the present day. The traditional foundryman practicing his profession as a craft, continues to produce, sell and export castings of considerable complexity and high quality. We have master craftsmen producing very high quality castings. On the other hand, we have foundries based on processes using modern technology and equipment rather than based on pure manual skills and ingenuity. There are foundries in India which have the technology and equipment comparable to most modern foundries of the world. Carrying this mixed bag of skill and learning, foundry industry has made great strides in the post-independent India. Earlier, a few decades ago, there were hardly any foundry equipment manufactured in the country and used to be imported. But, today, India can supply practically all needs of plant and machines for a modern medium sized mechanized foundry.[140] Sophisticated equipment such as Electric Arc and Induction Furnaces, Pressure Die Casting Machines, etc. are now being manufactured in India. Cupolas of international design and of capacities of 10 tonnes per hour or more are now manufactured in the country. All kinds of oil-fired and gas-fired and reverberatory melting furnaces and modern moulding machines are manufactured here.

The country has around 5000 foundries widely spread over the country producing 3.5 million metric tonnes of grey iron, ductile iron, steel and non-ferrous castings annually. The turnover of these foundries in the country reached an all-time height of Rs. 13, 000 crores ($ 3 billion) and export touched Rs. 16, 00 crores ($

0.35 billion) in the year 2002-03[139]. The bulk of these castings are that of gray iron (~74%), followed by steel castings (~10%), ductile iron (~8%) and rest aluminium and other non-ferrous castings. Similar figures for total casting production was 4.08 million tonnes of value of Rs. 15, 000 crores ($ ~ 3.5 billion) and exports of the order of 2000 crores ($ 0.46 billion) during 2003-2004.[141] It is expected that by 2007-08, India will produce 5.5 million tonnes of castings and export may rise to 5000 crores rupees. India will thus become foundry Giant and a Global Hub for international casting buyers.

16.3 IMPACT OF ECONOMIC REFORM POLICY AND GLOBILIZATION

The recent changes which have taken place in economic scenario and progressive government policies have made great impact on Indian foundry industry. As a result of Government's economic reform policy, internationalization of market place, improved communications and increasing awareness of quality, a technoeconomic upheaval is taking place in Indian foundry industry. Leading industrial giants from world over are now coming to India to either source their components or for setting up joint ventures. Traditional techniques have started giving way to new technology, tools, processes, equipment, mechanization and automation, non-destructive testing, inspection and quality control. Most of the current technological developments taking place have been a blending of technologies to suit Indian conditions and also blending of sophisticated foundry equipment with Indian equipments available. Some of the new developments are[139] converting the liquid pig iron directly into castings, use of high pressure moulding and latest moulding and core making processes using chemically bonded sands, installation of long campaign cupolas to give non-stop liquid metal for a week, use of continuous mixer, use of lost foam technology, etc. For these, several foreign companies of USA, UK, Germany, Japan and Belgium are collaborating with Indian foundries for providing technical know-how and financial assistance. Most Indian foundries are trying for the export market and also for the automobile market. Today, the Indian foundry industry, although beset with many problems, is facing foreign competition for taking over a significant portion of the global demand for value added castings in the automobile, machine tools, cement construction and engineering industry.

Some 400 of the Indian foundries have acquired quality certification of ISO9001 and 10 foundries in the country have a scale of production comparable to the biggest in the world. By 2004-05, at least 1000 foundries are expected to have got quality accreditation.

To meet the exacting demand of its global and domestic clientele, the Indian foundry has come a long way and taken bold decisions to modernize the infrastructure facilities in terms of melting, moulding, tool development, quality system etc. As mentioned earlier as well as to add further, some of the major steps taken by the Indian foundries are transition from Cupola to Duplexing/Induction-Melting leading to improved metallurgy of cast irons manufactured and from Jolt-Squeeze moulding process to high pressure moulding for better dimensional control and higher productivity, development of pattern and die with CAD/CAM. Process, increased awareness on quality systems, automation undertaken to eliminate hazardous operations, core making with Hot Box and Cold Box Processes and commitment to pollution control-ISO14000.[141] In efforts to boost casting production, foundry parks and clusters are being set up in some parts of the country.[145] Foundries in such clusters will have the scope to interact amongst themselves and pool resources for mutual benefit. They may secure common facilities for pollution monitoring and control of molten metal requirements, pattern equipment design and manufacture, moulding and core sand procurement and preparation, fettling, machining and finishing and marketing besides some administrative facilities such as security, transport and maintenance etc. A very common facility which could be profitably used is a robust training, testing, research and development unit.

16.4 PRESENT STATUS OF CAST IRON FOUNDRY PRACTICE

The cast iron foundry industry in India accounts for the largest tonnage of the cast metals produced (more than 80% of the cast metals produced are those of cast irons) and therefore largest number of foundries in this country are those of iron castings.

They are widely spread in the country but most of these foundries are situated in Agra, Batala, Ludhiana, Kolhapur, Belgaum, Pune, Bombay, Ahmedabad, Baroda, Rajkot, Jabalpur, Howrah, Kolkata, Coimbatore, Hyderabad, Bangalore and Chennai. A large number of these foundries (some 80%) are small and medium enterprises (SMEs) although there are a few foundries which compare to the most modern and biggest in the world.

These foundries can be grouped in various categories of the Gray Iron Foundries, White and Malleable Iron Foundries, S.G. Iron Foundries and Alloy Iron Foundries and their foundry practice can be discussed under the above headings as follows. The various foundry operation information and data given here are based on the author's collection from publications of Indian Foundry Journals, Indian Foundry Directories, his personal visits to few typical foundries and some report obtained from private communications[141-143].

16.4.1 Gray Iron Foundry Practice

Majority of the iron foundries in the country are those of gray iron and various common cast products of these foundries are manhole covers, C.I. pipes and fittings, water pumps, electric motors, brake drums, fly wheels, tractor parts, bearing covers, pulleys, heat exchanger parts, sugarmill parts, ingot mould, castings for agriculture sector such as diesel engines, rice and dal mill castings, gear box, pistons, crank case, cylinder liners, cylinder heads and blocks. Practically all grades of gray irons are produced and the size of the product widely varies in the range of a few kgs to as large as 50 tonnes. Barring a few small foundries, the annual turnover varies in the range of 2500 tonnes upto 90, 000 tonnes. The gray iron casting production has increased in the country from 2.4 to 2.84 million tonnes from 1999 to 2003 and it is expected that its production will still continue to increase to meet the increased demand of castings in the coming future.

Melting Practice: The cold-blast acid-lined conventional cupolas which are intermittently poured are invariably used is most gray iron foundries for melting. Cupolas of 24 to 60 inch internal diameters with melting capacity of 1 to 6 tonnes per hour are in common use. In some small foundries, cupolas are operated once or twice in a week with a melting campaign of 6 to 8 hours duration.

However, continuous cupolas with larger output of 10 to 20 tons per hour are also in use in some modern foundries. Besides conventional cupolas, divided blast and hot blast cupolas are also in operation and are used where a high degree of superheat is required. Gas-fired coke-less cupolas are also in operation on experimental basis, particularly in Agra regions.

In addition to cupolas, many foundries also use electric melting furnaces such as coreless medium or mains frequency induction furnaces and direct electric are furnaces as primary melting furnaces. The latter are available in foundries which also make steel castings. The core type induction holding furnaces are also in use for making bigger castings. The new foundries now prefer to go for electric melting as it provides a much cleaner and controlled melting. Before pouring, inorder to ensure a good cast structure (having A type of graphite flakes), some modern foundries add inoculants (FeSi or calcium silicide) to the melt in the range of 0.15 to 0.5% by weight of the melt.

Duplex melting practice such as cupola + rotary furnace or cupola + induction furnace melting is also adopted. Normally, a pouring temperature range of 1250 to 1450° C is employed depending upon the composition, section thickness and size of the casting poured. The melting charge meterial consists of foundry grade pig iron (PI), steel and cast iron scrap and gray iron foundry returns.

Moulding, Coremaking and Casting Practice: Gray iron castings are produced by almost all processes of casting available such as sand casting, permanent mould casting, centrifugal casting, etc. Among the sand casting processes, green sand moulding, dry sand moulding, core sand moulding using no-bake processes, CO_2 sand moulding, shell moulding and high pressure moulding are adopted. For economic reasons, however, green sand moulding is most often adopted.

The green moulding sand mixtures used have sufficient clay to provide high compression and shear strengths. It has also sufficient moisture to activate the bentonite (used as binder) and provide good permeability. Both the sodium-base and calcium-base bentonites or their combinations are used. Additives like sea coal, coke, graphite, pitch, etc. are also used to produce a reducing atmosphere in the mould for preventing oxidation of the metal and also to provide better surface finish (carbon used as mould coating). Use of wood, cereals or oat hulls, etc. is also made along with sea coal to accommodate sand expansion and provide better stripping characteristics.

The following is the typical composition of the green sand mixtures used depending on size of the casting:

Natural silica sand with GFN	:	60 to 75
Clay content	:	3 to 6%
Moisture content	:	2.5 to 4%
Volatile combustible matter such as coal dust	:	1 to 5%

Many foundries use natural silica sand and molasses as its binder. Synthetic sands using washed silica sands and controlled amounts of water and bentonites are also used for special casting purposes.

Dry sand moulding, shell moulding, CO_2-sand moulding or no-bake sand processes using furane resins or alcid 3 part systems are also adopted where greater strength and better permeability of the moulds are required. For good surface finish, graphite or zircon sand coating is also used.

A typical dry sand mixture may have the following composition:

Bentonite	:	1.5 to 2%
Dextrine	:	1 to 1.5%
Molasses	:	1%

For core making, all the available processes are in use such as oil, molasses and CO_2 sands, air-setting (no-bake) sands using phenolic resins, shell moulding sand, and cold and hot box sands.

A variety of pattern materials such as wooden pattern, aluminium patterns, thermocoal patterns or reinforced composite patterns (thermocoal reinforced with wood) are adopted for mould making. Floor and pit moulding, double box and flaskless moulding are in common practice for preparation of moulds. Besides manual moulding and core making, machine moulding processes using jolt-squeeze machines (most frequently used ones) are in common use. Many modern foundries also use high pressure moulding to obtain greater hardness and better dimensional control. In addition to manual sand preparation, many foundries also have semi-mechanized or fully mechanized sand preparation units. The shot blasting machine is also used for removal of sand and cleaning of the castings in addition to wire brushing, hand chipping, and pedestal grinders which are commonly used in many small foundries.

In addition to sand casting practice, the permanent mould casting is also employed for making small sized gray iron castings weighing less than 10 kg. This process is suitable for producing pressure castings such as castings for compressors and hydraulic cylinders. The centrifugal casting of gray irons using horizontal axis casting machines is also employed for making cast iron pipes and other circular and spherical products.

Some gray iron castings are given stress relieving treatment besides a few castings which are subjected to full annealing treatment.

16.4.2 White and Malleable Iron Foundry Practice

The production of the malleable castings in the country was of the order of 0.04 million tonnes during 2003-04 and it is expected that like the world trend, its production will decline due to its replacement by S.G. iron castings.

The production malleable iron requires first making of white iron casting which is mainly used for this purpose. The white iron is a very hard and brittle substance and therefore its other applications are those which require greater wear and abrasion resistance in the service such as bearings and spacer tools in form machinery, tumbling and pulverizing mill liners or crushing plants, hammers and parts of the ceramic industry. Chilled cast irons are also produced for applications requiring higher abrasive resistance on wearing surfaces such as grain mill rolls. However, as mentioned earlier, the main application of white iron casting is to serve as the feed material for the malleabilizing process for production of the malleable castings. The principal users of the malleable castings are the automotive and truck industries, producers of the construction machineries and agricultural equipment makers. The size of the malleable iron castings produced in the country varies usually in the range of 0.5 to 100 kg and may be as large as 3000 kg. The foundries making such castings are small in number and their annual outputs are also comparatively small upto the extent of 3000 to 4000 tonnes.

Melting Practice: The iron produced is melted in induction furnaces (both mains and medium frequency furnaces), rotary oil fired furnaces or by duplex melting using cupola and induction furnaces. The charge material comprises of P.I., steel crap and malleable foundry returns.

Moulding, Core making and Casting Practice: The technology of moulding and core making used in malleable iron foundry in general is similar to that used for gray iron castings for similar sizes and quantity of the castings. In fact, many gray iron foundries also make malleable castings.

Since the white iron castings are susceptible to hot cracking, the internal cores used require to be highly collapsible. This is obtained using core sands incorporating organic binders such as core oil, no-bake air-setting resins, etc. Moulds are also produced in silicate bonded CO_2-sand or resin bonded shell mould sand. Sands used for making moulds are required to be more heat resistant because of higher pouring temperature used for malleable irons. Synthetic moulding sands are therefore generally used although some foundries use natural sands as well.

Malleabilizing Practice: Batch type heat treatment furnaces are commonly used for annealing white iron castings. These furnaces may be oil-fired, coal or gas fired. The electric heat treatment furnaces are also used. Usually, blackheart malleabilizing is practiced for producing ferritic grades of malleable iron castings. The pearlitic malleable iron castings are also produced using the conventional heat treatment cycles for applications requiring high strength and hardness.

16.4.3 S.G. Iron Foundry Practice

S.G. cast iron is a revolutionary engineering material among the family of cast irons and its demand and production is increasing throughout the world including India at a fast rate because of the fact that this material uniquely combines the process advantages of gray iron (i.e. low melting point, good fluidity and castability) and product advantages of steel (i.e. high strength, toughness, ductility, hot workability and hardenability). Its production in the country was 0.363 million tonnes during 2003-04 and as compared to other cast irons, its production has seen the highest growth rate from 235, 000 tonnes in 1999 to 363400 tonnes in 2003.[141] It is expected that keeping pace with the world trend, its demand and production in the country will continue to increase in coming future as well.

As mentioned earlier, S.G. iron castings have replaced gray iron and malleable iron castings in many applications. It has also replaced even the steel forgings in some applications. Its main applications are the spun pipes for transport of water, gas and petroleum products, automobile castings such as crank shafts, cylinder liners, piston rings and parts of the cars, trucks, tractors and other commercial vehicles. A considerable amount of S.G. iron castings are also used as metal working rolls, punch dies, sheet metal dies, gears, etc. besides its general engineering applications in iron and steel plants, railways and other fields.

The size of the S.G. iron castings produced in Indian foundries vary over a wide range from 1 to 850 kg and even may be as large as 5 to 12 tonnes. Most of the existing gray iron foundries also produce S.G. iron castings in addition to some foundries devoted only to production of S.G. iron and malleable iron castings.

Melting Practice: Because of the low phosphorus and sulfur contents desired in the base metal needed for magnesium treatment, Indian pig iron is not desirable as charge material for melting purposes. As such, synthetic base iron is produced by melting selected steel scrap, ductile foundry returns, a carburizing agent such as coke, graphite or coconut shell and other necessary alloy additions in induction furnaces, both of mains frequency and medium frequency. Duplex melting is also used in some foundries having cupolas along with induction furnaces or electric arc furnaces. In such cases, desulphurization of the iron produced is carried out outside in the ladles by treatment with lime, CaC_2 or soda ash. When induction furnaces are used as primary melting furnaces, they are usually in 2 to 6 in numbers with melting capacity of 1 to 3 tons, depending upon the production requirements. The pouring temperature of metal usually varies in the range of 1470 to 1500° C to take care of the loss in temperature during magnesium treatment in subsequent operation.

Moulding, Coremaking and Casting Practice: The technology of moulding and casting of S.G. iron castings is similar to that used for gray iron castings of similar size. The most common moulding and casting processes employed are green and dry sand moulding, shell moulding, CO_2-sand moulding, no-bake or air-setting sand moulding and centrifugal casting. The moulding sands used are also similar to those used in gray iron foundries but the moisture is strictly controlled to avoid oxidation of magnesium present in the melt. The combustible material in sands is also limited to 6 to 7%. Modern foundries use high pressure moulding to give dense and strong moulds capable of preventing mould wall movement. For core making, similar processes such as CO_2-sand, no-bake/air-setting sand and oil-sand process as used in gray iron foundries are commonly employed.

Magnesium Treatment: For spheroidization, the most universally used Magnesium Treatment method is adopted in all foundries. Magnesium-Ferrosilicon alloy containing small amount of magnesium (4 to 10% Mg) is used as the treatment agent. Various methods which are commonly adopted in different foundries for introducing the alloy in the molten base metal are:

1. Sandwich Process
2. Pour Over Method

Sandwich Process: In this method, the treatment alloy is placed into a recession in the bottom of the ladle. The alloy is then covered by a steel plate, sheet iron or iron chips or some inert material such as sand and then the metal is poured. In this way, the reaction time between the magnesium and the iron is delayed until the ladle is at least partially filled with the metal and thus increases the recovery of magnesium. Some foundries use a crude method of putting the alloy inside a steel box kept in the bottom of the ladle and then pouring the metal over it.

Pour Over Method: This is most commonly used method in which the treatment alloy is kept one side on the bottom of the ladle and the metal is poured into the opposite side of the bottom of the ladle so that it spreads slowly over the treatment alloy. In such cases, tall ladle with tundish cover is used. The tundish covers over the tall ladle such that metal falls into the opposite side of the ladle.

In addition to above methods, some modern foundries also use the famous American Magnesium Impregnated Coke Process in which the plunged treatment agent coming in contact with hot metal leads to slow evolution of the magnesium vapour from the pores of the coke. After the treatment, the coke floats easily on the surface of the metal and skimmed. This is a much cheaper process (as coke is used as the carrier agent) than the methods using specially prepared costly treatment alloys.

The treatment alloy used amounts to 0.5 to 2.5% of the melt weight. The treatment temperature and time also vary from 1450 to 1500° C and 20 seconds to 2 minutes, respectively.

Post Inoculation: There are variations in the methods adopted for the inoculation of the magnesium treated alloy. In one method, the usual inoculant (FeSi) is added into the metal stream while it is tapped into another ladle (Stream Inoculation) before pouring the moulds. In another method, the inoculant is added into the ladle containing half of the treated metal, mixing it well into melt and then adding the other half of the treated metal into the ladle. The weight of the inoculant added varies from 0.1 to 0.3% of the weight of the treated metal. The common grades of FeSi alloys containing 75 or 85% silicon is used as inoculant. Some foundries also use calcium-silicon alloy in place of FeSi.

After the post inoculation, the metal is poured into the moulds quickly. The pouring temperature varies over a range of 1260° C to 1410° C.

After the solidification of the casting, it is separated and cleaned using the conventional methods adopted in the gray iron foundries. Sand blasting machines are also used in some modern foundries.

Heat Treatment: S.G. iron castings are used as-cast in some cases. However, stress relieving treatment is usually given in most foundries before it is supplied to customers. Some castings may be heat treated by annealing, normalizing or by quenching and tempering depending on specific property requirements.

16.4.4 Alloy Iron Foundry Practice

As such, there is hardly any exclusive Alloy Iron Foundry for making alloy iron castings. They are usually a part of the S.G. Iron or Malleable Iron foundries devoted to production of such castings. Among the alloy irons, Ni-Hard and Ni-Resist iron castings are usually made. Standard grades of Ni-Hard iron castings are used for applications such as grinding rolls, ball and tumbling mill liners and rolls for steel mills. Ni-resist iron castings are heat-and corrosion-resistant castings and are used for pump parts, boiler fittings and parts for handling of acids and alkalies. The castings prepared in Indian foundries vary in size range from 1 to 500 kg.

Melting Practice: For melting of these alloy irons, induction furnaces or electric arc furnaces are commonly used. Acid lined furnaces are used as they are economical and require little adjustments to slag compositions. Normal charge materials are various kinds of steel scrap, foundry returns of similar alloys. High-carbon ferrochrome is used for alloying iron with chromium. Nickel may be obtained from the foundry returns of similar alloy and/or nickel shots generally added near the end of the heat to avoid excessive oxidation losses. Carbon is obtained from electrode graphite or other sources. Silicon and manganese are added as ferro alloys. High superheating temperatures are not necessary when electric melting furnaces like induction or arc furnaces are used. Metal is poured at a temperature range of 1450 to 1550° C.

Moulding, Coremaking and Casting Practice: Ni-Hard alloys may be sand-cast or chill-cast in permanent moulds depending upon hardness required. For making sand moulds, green sand, dry sand, oil-sand, no-bake sands, shell mould and CO_2-sands are employed. Similar sands (except the green sands) are also used for coremaking. Centrifugal casting is also adopted for making circular or spherical shapes of the products.

Heat Treatment: Above alloy castings are usually given stress relieving treatments to relieve the casting stresses. Annealing of some casting may be necessary to reduce the hardness. In case of Ni-Hard alloys, tempering is performed between 205 to 260° C for at least 4 hours to temper the martensite structure and increase the strength and toughness as may be required in some applications.

There are hardly any foundry in the country which produces Vermicular or Compacted Graphite Iron castings and this material is still in the state of R & D in various laboratories of the academic institutions and national research laboratories.

16.5 PROBLEMS FACED BY IRON FOUNDRIES AND THEIR POSSIBLE SOLUTIONS

Although Indian cast iron foundry industry has made rapid strides in the recent past year, there are still certain basic problems faced by this industry. These problems need to be solved not only to make these iron foundries becoming competitive in the world trade and grab a large portion of the export market, but also enable them to meet the ever increasing domestic demands of the various engineering industries. Some of the major problems being faced by the cast iron foundry industry and their possible remedies are:

1. Non-availability of supply of basic raw materials both in quantity and quality as well as in time is a major bottle neck in cast iron foundries. It is obvious from the data given in preceding sections that gray iron castings constitute the largest tonnage of the castings produced by the Indian foundries. The cupola is the main melting unit of such iron foundries and the pig iron, coke and scrap (steel and cast iron scrap) are the main raw materials needed for the same. The present scenario of supply of these basic materials are as follows.

   Pig Iron: The current demand of foundry grade pig iron (PI) in the country is about 2 million tonnes[144] all of which is presently being met by secondary PI producers as after liberalization 21 new blast furnaces with a capacity of about 3.9 million tonnes have been permitted to be installed out of which 16 units are commissioned increasing total production of PI from 1.6 million tonnes in 1991-92 to 5.28 million tonnes in 2002-03. During 2003-04, production of PI was 5.22 million tonnes of which 0.971 million tonnes came from main producers (steel plants) and 4.25 million tonnes was made available from secondary producers[144]. However, of this, the foundry grade PI as demanded by the cast iron industry was about 2 million tonnes. The main producers of PI (steel plants) normally supply basic grades of PI which is suitable for steel making only. The present demand of foundry grade pig iron has considerably increased over the earlier figures and thus supply of this basic raw material has become scarce both in quantity and quality. The solution could be whether our country should import PI from country like Brajil or China.

   The global price trend of PI is that it is continually increasing and the supply of PI from China is becoming scarce and expensive[145]. For this, Indian Government should negotiate a barter deal with China offering iron ore against supply of PI as well as coal/coke needed by the industry. The Government should also reduce the import duty of PI to have control on the price rise of PI and should persuade the steel plants to increase the supply of P.I. to foundry industry by exclusively reserving their one or two blast furnaces for making and supplying the foundry grade pig iron to cast iron industry only.

Further, the Indian P.I. which is available has relatively high phosphorus and sulfur and is therefore, not suitable for production of S.G. and malleable iron castings. Although the sulfur content can be kept down to the required limit by external desulphurization, we still need to produce synthetic iron compositions by melting selected steel scrap and adding necessary carburizer in electric furnaces, particularly to meet the composition need of S.G. iron castings.

Coke: Non-availability of suitable coke is another most important factor affecting cupola operation. Indian coke has very high ash content which adversely influences the combustibility of coke, melting efficiency and hence, the smooth and efficient operation of the cupola. Usually, a large size hard coke is required for efficient cupola operation. Thus, in practice, Indian foundries use whatever grade of coke is available besides their high prices. The coke, therefore, needs to be imported.

The cost of imported coke however has increased considerably in recent years and thus it has also become scarce. Many PI manufactures have therefore switched over to using coal as raw material instead of coke[144]. Further, Indian coals are also high in ash and therefore low-ash coals are required to be imported. The available deposits of domestic high-ash coking coals are also controlled by the government related agencies. Moreover, the existing coke ovens in the country are technologically backward resulting in high cost of coke production and poor quality which in turn lead to higher coke consumption for PI manufacture. Thus, again here, the Indian Government has to sort out the problems which are under their commands and should help in importing coke/coal while making deal with foreign countries like China for import of PI.

Scrap: The other major raw material is the scrap which also needs to be imported to meet the present demand both in quantity and quality and this again depends on the foreign supplies and their prices prevailing. There has been abnormal increase in the prices of steel scrap, ferro-alloys like PI. The question is whether there is any other alternative material for this like sponge iron which is being produced in the country by direct reduction processes. This should be explored.

Hence, in general, the Government policies are required to be made to enable global procurement of all above vital raw materials needed by the cast iron foundry industry to help them compete globally, both commercially and technically.

2. It is true that Indian foundries have blend of both old and modern foundries and a large percentage of these foundries is in the small sector and many of them can still be considered to be obsolete in terms of modern foundry technology. Most of the iron foundries in Agra and other regions are examples of such foundries.[143] The use of obsolete and primitive technology in such foundries result in low productivity, wastage of material, lower quality of the product and unfavourable working conditions. There is thus urgent and pressing needs to upgrade the existing technology, equipment and operating practices in these foundries which are today still working under backyard conditions. Also, indigenous know-how and process details are required to be developed to utilize new technology and equipment.
3. There is dearth of people who have the right kind of training to respond to the needs of changing foundry industry in the country. A very alarming situation exists in the country in this context that a large number of cast iron foundries hire labour on the contract basis from the Mistries or other local agents and get the entire technical work done by them instead of using their own regular employees who may have the right kind of qualification and training to produce the quality products. This situation should be immediately tackled by the appropriate authorities and the foundry work

should be carried out with the help of regular employees only. However, even these employees also need to undergo continuous training and their skill should be upgraded to cope-up with the needs of modern foundry practice. Not only the labourer, but even the supervisory staff and the management also need proper training for optimum utilization of available resources of men, machines, material and money. Particularly, the management staff, should be deputed to attend the seminars/conferences held in the areas of cast iron technology to keep abreast of the latest developments taking place in this field and take necessary steps to adopt them for their foundries to improve the quality of the products as well as the productivity. They should have increased awareness on quality systems and should learn to introduce techniques like 6 Sigma, TQM, TPM, etc. for optimum utilization of resources available.

4. Keeping pace with the world trend, many of the present iron foundries and particularly, the new installations are going for more and more electric melting systems as they are clean, more controllable and lead to least air pollution. As such, a large number of existing Indian foundries have electric induction and arc melting furnaces as their melting units. One major problem of such foundries is the non-availability of sufficient and uninterrupted supply of quality electric power at reasonable price. This mainly leads to poor or partial utilization of the installed capacity of the foundry units. A recent survey shows that the capacity utilization of Agra based foundry units due to power cuts is of the order of 15 to 20% only as against an all India average of about 50%.[143] There is thus need to generate more electric power and distribute it properly so that all Indian foundries are capable of utilizing their full installed capacities. The Government should help in this respect and captive power generation should be encouraged with no tax levied on such power generation.
5. As mentioned earlier, a number of foundries have very bad working conditions as no measures or insufficient measures have been taken to tackle the pollution problems of their foundries. All kinds of pollution take place including

emissions and fumes from melting furnaces in the presence of which employees have to work which is very unhygienic situation. There is thus pressing need to install proper air pollution control equipments including the pollution monitoring and measuring systems. The fume extraction hoods atleast should be installed above the moulds poured with molten metal. Besides fumes and heats, workers also suffer from noise pollution. One simple step could be to isolate fettling stations outside the main foundry bay to reduce noise and dust.

6. For modernization and expansion of the existing iron foundry units, finance is the vital input required. The Government and other finance agencies should effort not only to make finance easily available to them but also at reasonable rates.

It is therefore necessary that these major problems should be solved with priority to further improve the turnover and quality of the iron castings to meet the present and future demands of the country.

16.6 FUTURE NEEDS AND CHALLANGES

The cast iron foundry industry has a major role to play in the economic development of our country. It has been felt by our planners in this industry that upgradation of the technology is now the only answer to our becoming competitive in the world market. To be successful global player, we need to upgrade technology in some of the areas and bring in the modern foundry equipment and employ computers for designing, process control and foundry management. It is a matter of pleasure that to meet the exacting demand of its global and domestic, clientele, the cast iron industry has come along way and has taken some bold decisions to modernize the infrastructure facilities interms of melting, moulding, coremaking, tool development and quality systems.

This will result in production of quality castings meeting international standards at competitive prices. However, it is also necessary to bring our industry closer to the international market. Today, all our customers are demanding timely delivery and quality product at very competitive price and the industry has to adhere to it. In the context of the globalization, cast iron industry has to face the change in quality, price and delivery schedule of the product in the open market trend. There is urgent need to cast to global standards by producing high quality castings complying with ISO standards. This will help Indian foundries to grab a major portion of the world market and hence, contribute significantly towards the economic growth of the country.

There is a reasonable projection that, by 2010, ferrous casting production in India will double to around 6 million tonnes[140]. Thus there is very excellent business opportunity for the Indian foundries to sell their products in the world market besides meeting the domestic demands. Some of the world giants are very keen to source their requirements from India because of high cost in their countries, their heavy expenditure on pollution control measures and also because of the reluctance of their younger engineering force to work in a foundry. Fortunately, our country is a labour intensive country and our foundry people are a tougher lot with strong will-power to sail through all odds and survive. Our foundry industry also has a large base spread across the country and we can meet the requirement of skilled manpower at low cost. Our country is also strategically best located for export. We therefore need to exploit these advantages to grab such export orders. All these will ultimately lead to a large expansion of the existing cast iron foundry units as well installation of many new ventures which will inturn help to solve the persisting unemployment problem of the country to a great extent.

In view of the strong competition being faced from some foreign countries like China, Korea and Taiwan, we now need to prepare a road-map to be globally competitive such as adding value by supplying machined castings from a single source, adhering strictly to delivery schedule, reducing development lead-times, continuously improving productivity and quality to reduce unit cost of the product, etc.[146] Our mission should be to make India a world foundry base and best casting supplier to global industry and for this, we need to design our strategy, understand our competitive advantages and ways to exploit it. It will be worthwhile to quote here a few sentences taken from the address delivered[147] by Mrs. Prabha Kulkarni, Ex-President, Institute of Indian Foundrymen during 50th Indian Foundry Congress held at Goa that "From time immemorial, it has been amply proved that we Indians are fast learners with a strong quest for acquiring knowledge and competent enough to face any challenge and any technical revolution that come our way". Thus, there is all the hope that people of our present cast iron industry will come up to meet the expectations as out lined above and hence, contribute significantly towards the economic growth of the country.

References

61. R. B. Gundlach, *Metals Handbook,* Vol. 15, Casting, ASM International, 1988 p. 678.
62. G. V. Challam and A. Anjaneyulu, Procd. Seminar on Cast Iron Today, Feb. 21-22, 1970, Bombay, IIF, p. 44.
63. R. B. L. Bharadwaj, ibid, p. 73.
64. F. Maratray, Trans. AFS, 1971, Vol. 79, p. 121.
65. W. Fairhurst and K. Rohrig, *Foundry Trade J.*, 1974, Vol 96, p. 271.
66. R. B. Gundlach, *Metals Handbook,* Vol. 15, Casting, ASM International, 1988, p. 699.
67. P. M. Bhagwati and N. Rama Murthi, Procd. Seminar on Cast Iron Today, Feb. 21-22, 1970, Bombay, IIF, p. 85.
68. H. T. Angus, *Cast Iron—Physical and Engineering Properties*, Butterworth, London, 1978, p. 223.
69. E. C. Rollason, *Metallurgy for Engineers*, Edward Arnold P. Ltd., Hill Street, 1973, p. 280.
70. V. G. S. Mani and P. S. Seshadri, Procd. Seminar on Cast Iron Today, Feb. 21-22, 1970, Bombay, IIF, p. 97.
71. R. B. Gundlach, *Metals Handbook,* Vol. 15, Casting, ASM International, 1988, p. 701.
72. R. Schneidwind and R. G. McElwee, Trans. AFS, Vol. 58, 1950, p. 65.
73. H. T. Anqus, D. Marles and M. H. Hilman, *BCIRA Journal*, Vol. 6, 1955, p. 201.
74. C. F. Walton, *The Gray Iron Castings Handbook,* Gray Iron Founders Society.
75. H. T. Anqus, *Cast Iron—Physical and Engineering Properties*, Butterworth, London, 1978.
76. B. C. Sastry, Procd. Seminar on Cast Iron Today , Feb 21-22, 1970, Bombay IIF, p. 149-172.
77. R. L. Hancher, *Brit Foundrym.*, 1963, Vol. 56, p. 375.
78. R. L. Hancher, ibid, 1969, Vol. 62, p. 38.
79. S. N. Mookerji and J. C. Kapur, Procd. Seminar on Cast Iron Today, Feb. 21-22, Bombay, IIF, p. 239-246.

80. S. P. Sharma, ibid, p. 212-214.
81. M. C. Agrawal and D. V. Paranjpe, TISCO, Vol. 8, 1962, p. 72.
82. Procd. of Seminar on Cast-Iron Today, Feb. 21-22, 1970, Bombay, IIF Publication, p. 201.
83. S. N. Tiwari, A. K. Ghosh and S. L. Malhotra, *Ind. Foundry, J.*, Vol. 24, 1978, p. 21.
84. C. S. Sivaram Krishnan, ibid., Vol. 48, No. 1, 2002, p. 46.
85. K. V. Sai Srinath, ibid., Vol. 52, No. 10, 2006, p. 39.
86. Welding Handbook, Section-4, America Welding Society, pp. 62-1.
87. H. T. Angus, *Cast Iron—Physical & Engineering Properties*, Butterworth, London, 1978, p. 382.
88. Ravi Menon, *Metals Hand Book*, Vol. 15, Casting, ASM International, 1988, p. 520.
89. F. A. Ball and D. R. Thorneycroft, *Foundry Tr. J.*, 1954, Vol. 97, p. 499.
90. G. R. Pease, *Weld J.*, 1960, Vol. 39, p. 1.
91. R. L. Kumar, Foundry, 1968, Vol. 96, p. 64.
92. C. Cookson, *Met. Constr. Br. Weld. J.*, 1971, Vol. 3, No. 5, p. 179.
93. R. A. Bishel, ibid. 1973, Vol. 5, p. 372.
94. C. Cookson, ibid, 1973, Vol. 5, p. 370.
95. A. G. Hogaboom, *Weld J.*, 1977, Vol. 56, p. 17.
96. S. D. Kiser, *Trans. AFS*, 1977, Vol. 85, p. 431.
97. R. Mohler, *Plant Eng.*, 1977, Vol. 31, p. 171.
98. J. H. Devletian, *Weld J.*, 1978, Vol. 57, p. 183.
99. E. H. La Grelins, *Trans. AFS*, 1947, Vol. 55, p. 375.
100. W. E. Thomas, ibid, 1947, Vol. 55, p. 482.
101. D. T. Martin, ibid, 1950, Vol. 58, p. 692.
102. K. M. Smith, ibid, 1951, Vol. 59, p. 304.
103. AFS Committee 66, ibid, 1962, Vol. 70, p. 1235.
104. P. J. Emerson, Procd. Seminar on Cast Iron Today, IIF, Bombay, 1970, p. 192.
105. R. W. Heine, C. R. Loper and P. C. Rosenthal, *Principles of Metal Casting*, Tata McGraw-Hill Publishing Co. Ltd., New Delhi, 1976, p. 682.
106. *ASM Hand Book*, Vol. 15, Casting, ASM International, 1988, pp. 544 to 556.
107. T. Marek, *Fundamentals in the Production & Design of Castings*, John Wiley & Sons, New York, 1956, pp. 313 & 335.
108. *Casting Design Hand Book*, ASM, Metals Park, Ohio, 1962, pp. 1-65.
109. *Cast Metals Hand Book*, AFS, Chicago, 1944, p. 18.
110. P. R. Beely, Foundry Technology, Butterworths/Heinemann, Oxford, 2001, p. 362.
111. L. Chapman, *Mod. Cast.*, 1966, Vol. 49, No. 3, p. 63 & Vol. 50, No. 7, p. 56.
112. R. M. Kotschi, *Metals Hand Book*, Vol. 15, Casting, ASM International, p. 598.
113. K. N. Kinkar, Procd. Seminar on Cast Iron Today, 1970, Bombay, IIF, p. 183.
114. R. W. Ruddle, Running and Gating of Sand Castings, Institute of Metals, London, 1956.
115. P. K. Sandell, *Indian Foundry J.*, 1969, No. 8, p. 105.

116. L. Smith, *British Foundrym*, 1976, No. 2, p. 44.
117. J. F. Wallace and E. B. Evans, *AFS Trans.*, 1957, Vol. 65, p. 267.
118. P. R. Beeley, *Foundry Technology*, 2nd edn., Butternorth/Heinemann, Oxford, 2001, p. 15.
119. H. W. Dietert, *Trans. AFS*, 1926, Vol. 34, p. 1038.
120. H. W. Dietert, *Foundry*, 1955, Vol. 81, No. 8, p. 205.
121. L. F. Porter and P. C. Rosenthal, *Trans. AFS*, 1952, Vol. 60, p. 725.
122. P. C. Mukherjee, *Fundamentals of Metal Casting Technology*, Oxford & IBH Publishing Co., New Delhi, 1979, p. 324.
123. C. F. Walton, *Foundry*, 1953, Vol. 81, No. 2, p. 100.
124. J. F. Wallace, ibid, 1959, Vol. 87, No. 11, p. 75.
125. H. D. Merchant, *Mod. Cast.*, 1959, Vol. 42, No. 2, p. 73.
126. J. Weston and V. Kondic, *Foundry Tr. J.*, 1961, Vol. 111, No. 2, p. 791.
127. V. Kondic, *Mod. Cast.*, 1965, Vol. 98, No. 7, p. 81.
128. J. F. Wallace and E. B. Evans, ibid, 1957, Vol. 40, No. 9, p. 47.
129. J. B. Caine, *AFS Trans.*, 1948, Vol. 56, p. 492.
130. H. F. Bishop, W. S. Pellini and E. T. Myskowski, ibid, 1955, Vol. 63, p. 271.
131. R. Wlodawer, *Directional Solidification of Steel Castings*, Pergamon Press, Oxford, 1966.
132. L. A. Plutshak and A. L. Suschil, *ASM Hand Book*, Vol. 15, Casting, ASM International, 2006, p. 577.
133. J. F. Wallace and E. B. Evans, *AFS Trans.*, 1958, Vol. 66, p. 49.
134. G. K. Turnbull, H. D. Merchant and J. F. Wallace, ibid, 1960, Vol. 68, p. 1.
135. I. C. H. Hughes, *ASM Hand Book*, Vol. 15, Casting, ASM International, 2006, p. 647.
136. R. A. Flinn, D. J. Reese and W. A. Spindler, *AFS Trans.*, 1955, Vol. 63, p. 720.
137. H. F. Bishop and W. S. Pellini, ibid, 1950, Vol. 58, p. 185.
138. M. Muralidhar and G. L. Datta, *Indian Foundry J.*, 2002, Vol. 48, No. 2, p. 26.
139. S. R. V. Ramanan, ibid., 2004, Vol. 50, No. 7, p. 6.
140. D. K. Seksaria, ibid., 2005, Vol. 51, No. 7, 2005, p. 41.
141. *Indian Foundry Directory*, 2005, p. 10.
142. *Indian Foundry Directory*, 2006, p. 33.
143. Report on Status of Foundry Industry at Agra, 2006, Private Communication.
144. Harsh Kumar and Rajesh Mishra, *Indian Foundry J.*, 2005, Vol. 51, No. 3, p. 33.
145. Editorial, ibid., 2004, Vol. 50, No. 3, p. 17.
146. Rajinder Malhar, ibid., 2005, Vol. 51, No. 3, p. 41.
147. Presidential Address, ibid., 2002, Vol. 48, No. 1, p. 17.

Subject Index

Author Index